Autism Spectrum Disorders - Advances at the End of the Second Decade of the 21st Century

Edited by Michael Fitzgerald

Published in London, United Kingdom

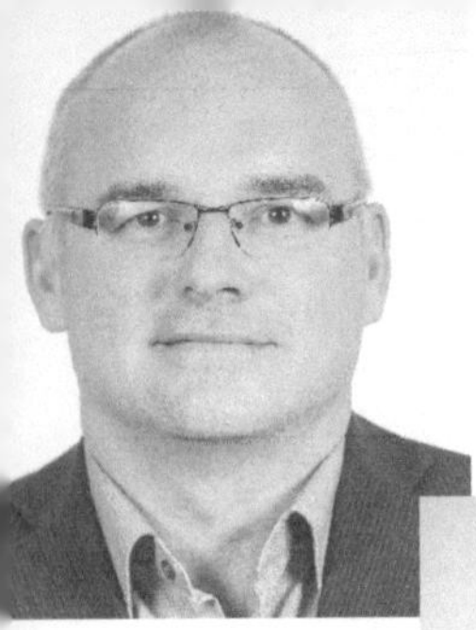
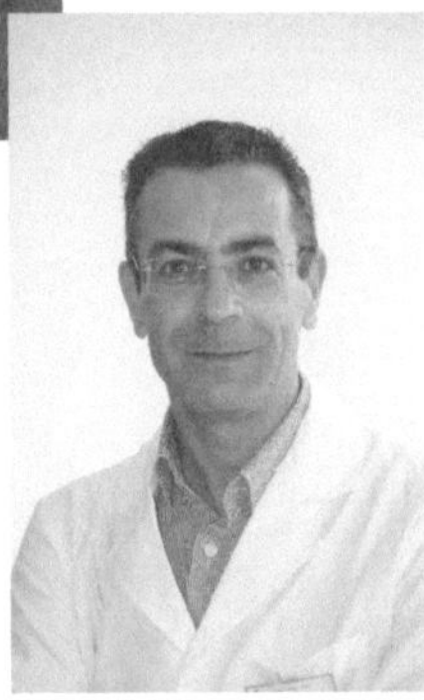
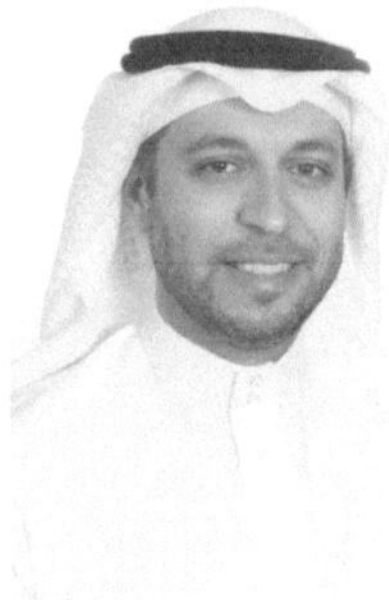
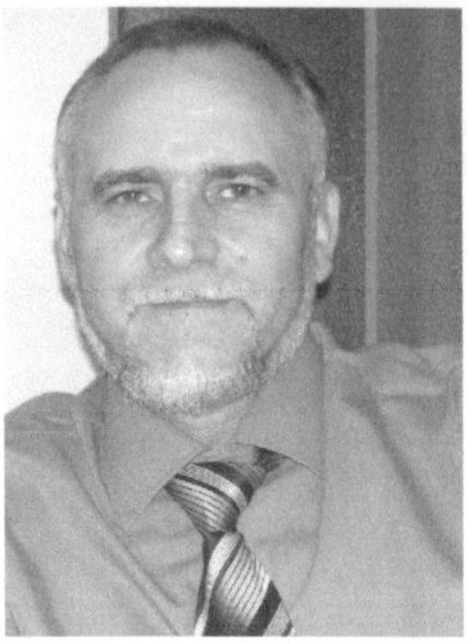
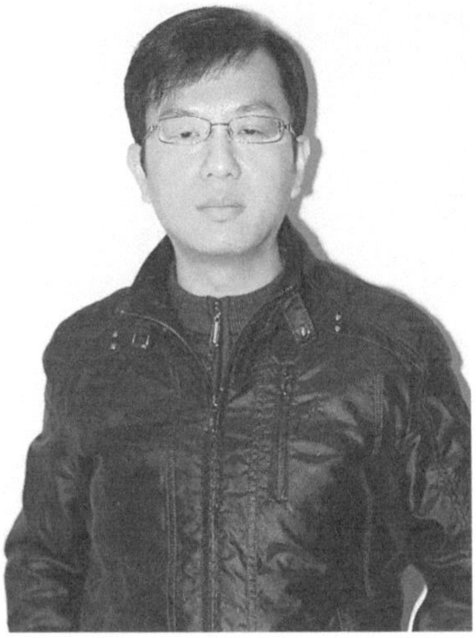
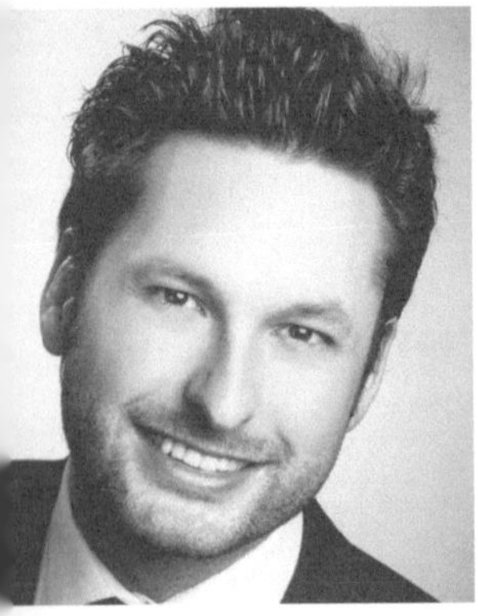
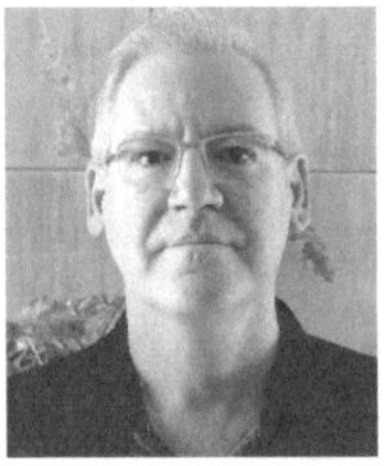

IntechOpen

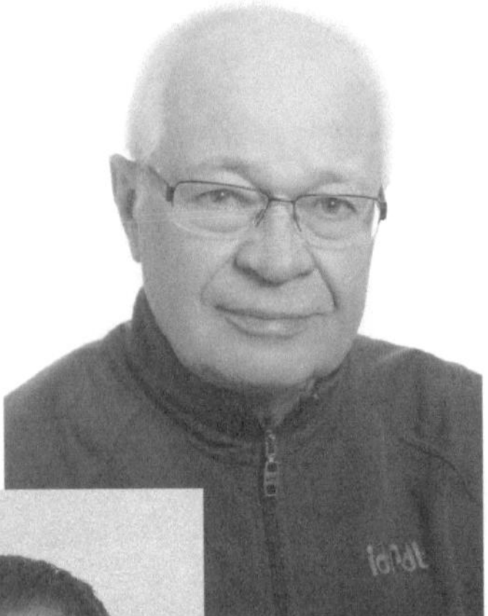
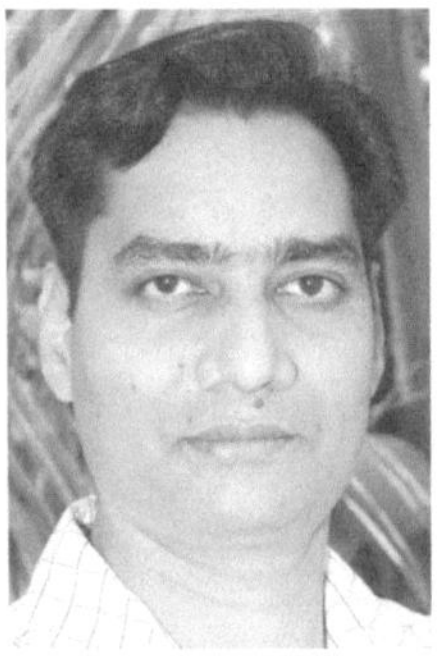
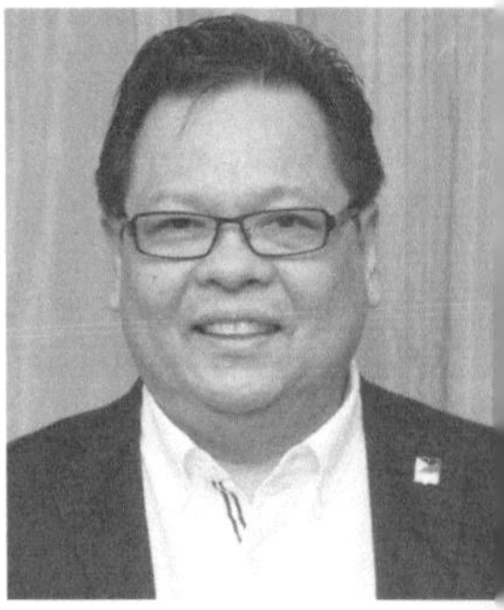
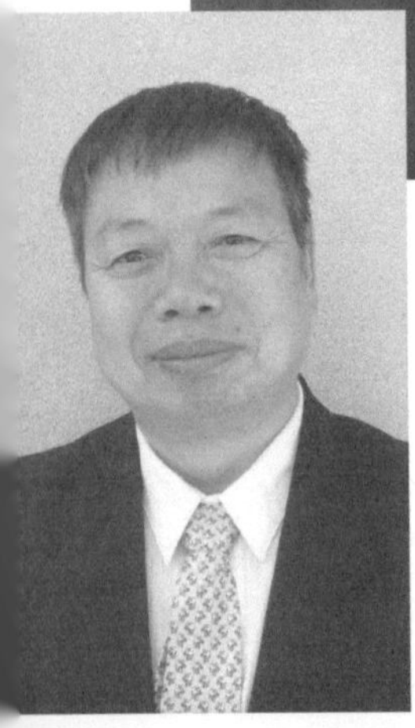
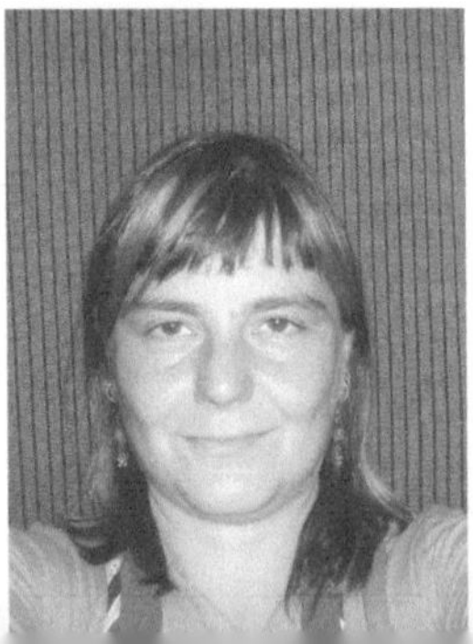
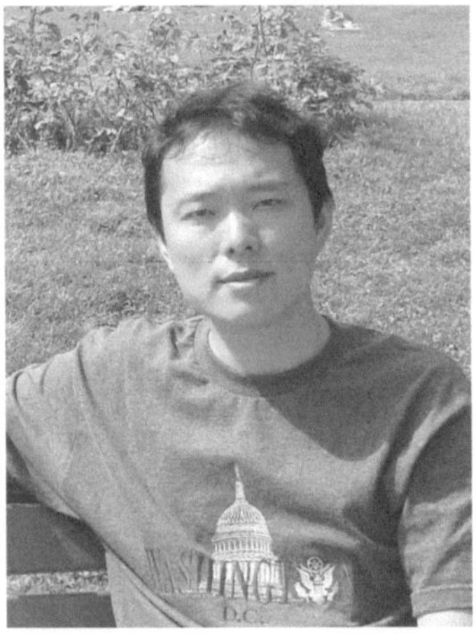

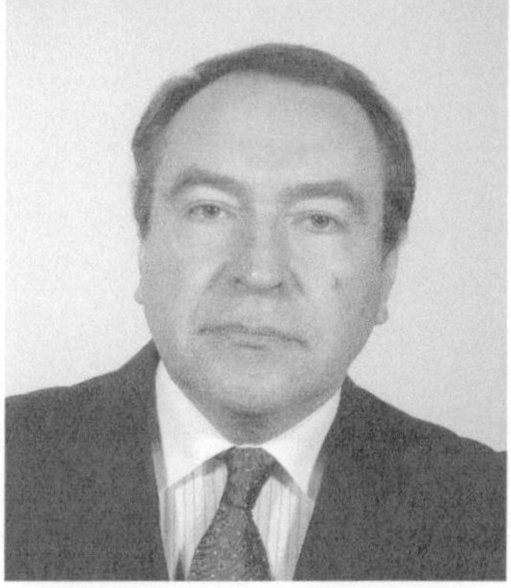
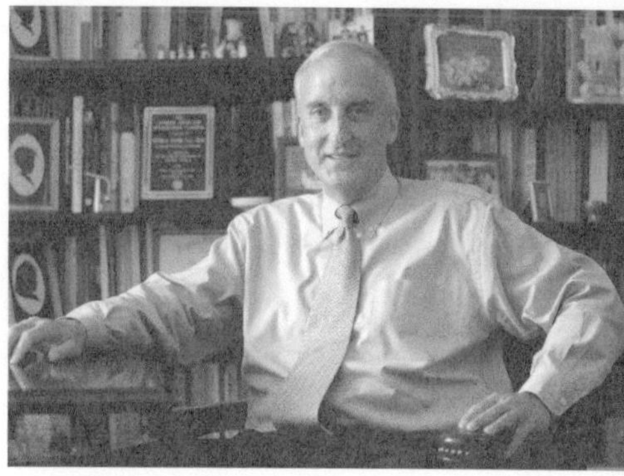
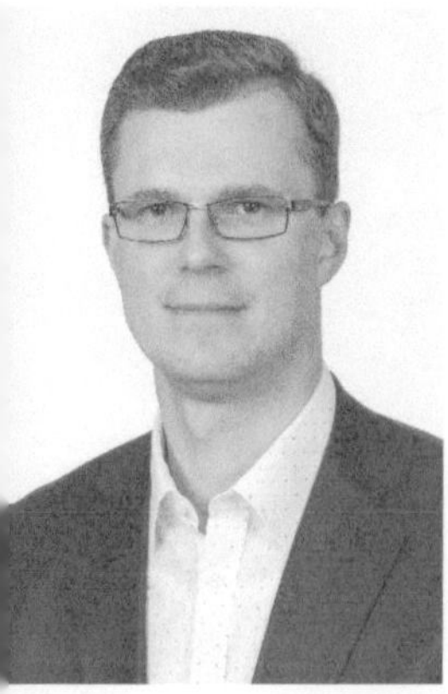
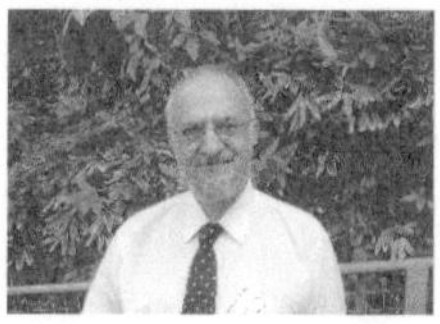
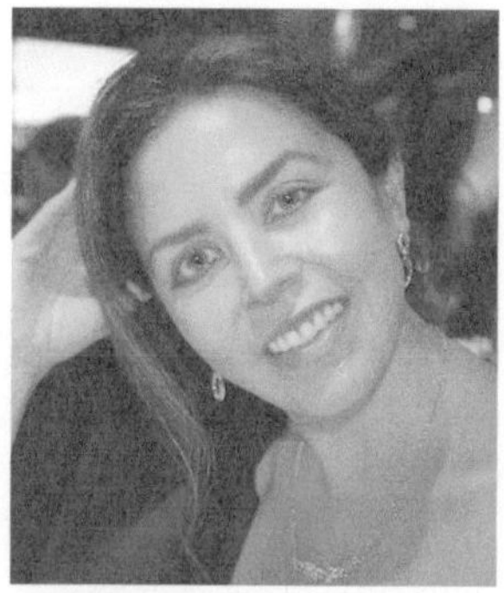

Supporting open minds since 2005

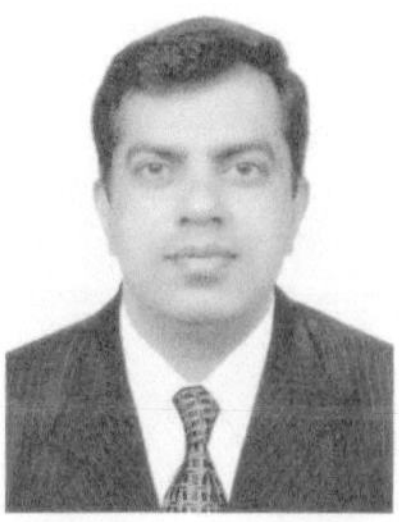
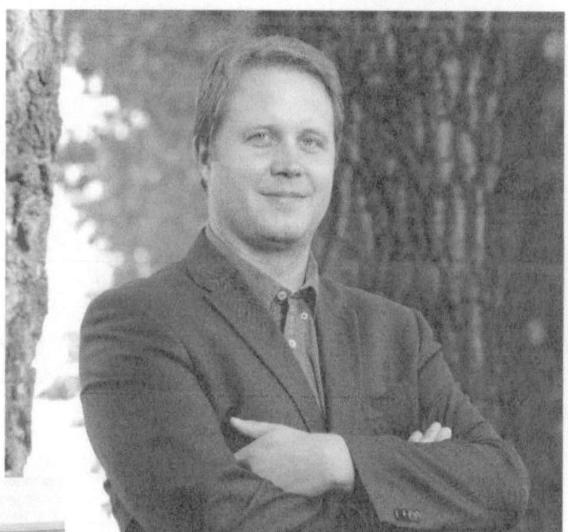
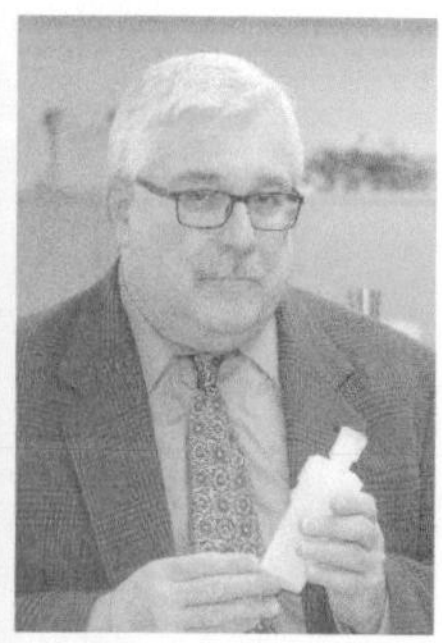
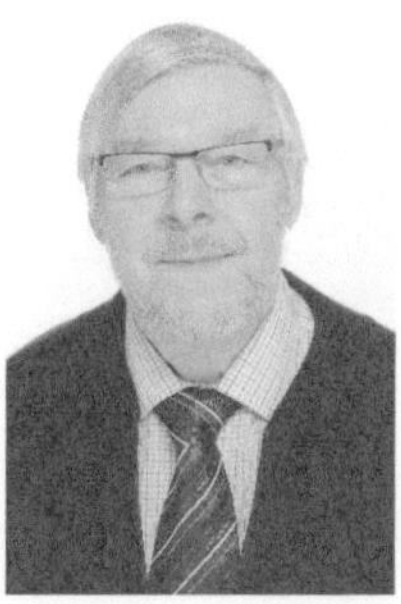
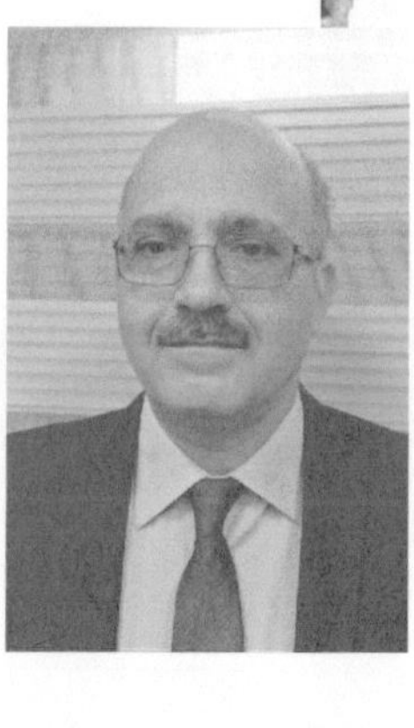
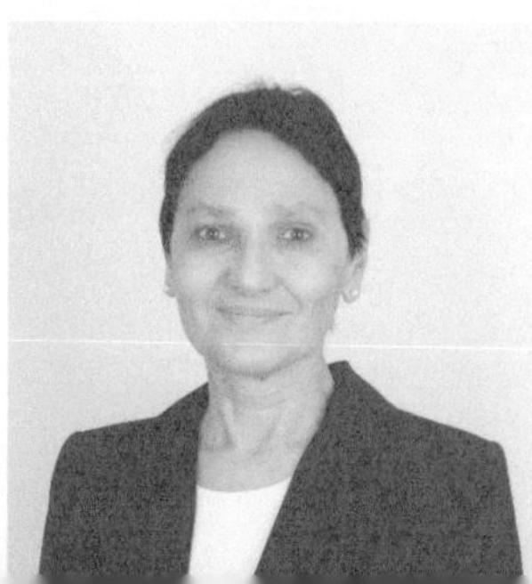
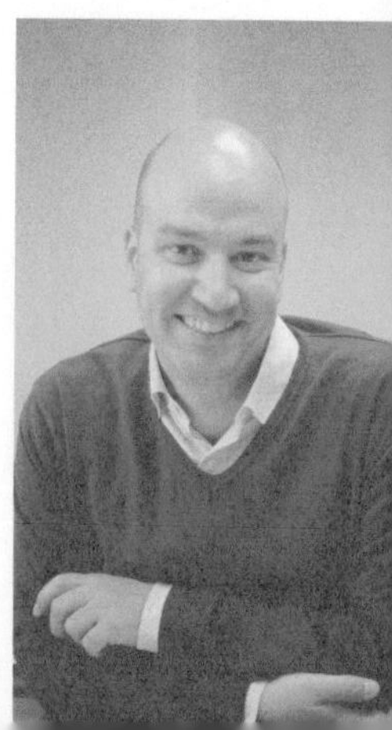

Autism Spectrum Disorders - Advances at the End of the Second Decade of the 21st Century
http://dx.doi.org/10.5772/intechopen.77652
Edited by Michael Fitzgerald

Contributors
David Kitara Lagoro, Denis Anywar Arony, Suzanne Gazda, Jan Blacher, Yasamine Bolourian, Katherine K.M. Stavropoulos, Chuen Heung Yau, Cheuk Long Ip, Yuk Yin Chau, Ho Cheung Lai, Troy D. Wood, Amber Flynn Charlebois, Emily R. Rose Sekera, Heather L. Rudolph, Christopher L. Pennington, Yong Seok Choi, Giuseppe Fanciulli, Michael Fitzgerald

First published in London, United Kingdom, 2019 by IntechOpen
IntechOpen is the global imprint of INTECHOPEN LIMITED, registered in England and Wales, registration number: 11086078, The Shard, 25th floor, 32 London Bridge Street
London, SE19SG - United Kingdom
Printed in Croatia

British Library Cataloguing-in-Publication Data
A catalogue record for this book is available from the British Library

Additional hard and PDF copies can be obtained from orders@intechopen.com

Autism Spectrum Disorders - Advances at the End of the Second Decade of the 21st Century
Edited by Michael Fitzgerald
p. cm.
Print ISBN 978-1-78984-021-6
Online ISBN 978-1-78984-022-3
eBook (PDF) ISBN 978-1-83962-273-1

Meet the editor

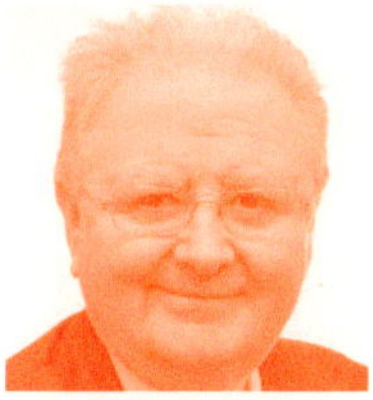

Professor Michael Fitzgerald was the first Professor of Child and Adolescent Psychiatry in Ireland. Specialising in autism spectrum disorders, he has diagnosed over 5000 sufferers. He has a large number of peer-reviewed publications and has written, co-written, and co-edited 34 books with Japanese, Dutch, and Polish translations. Professor Simon Baron-Cohen of the University of Cambridge described one of his books on autism as "the best book on autism" and described him as an "exceptional scholar." He has lectured extensively throughout the world, including the Royal Society/British Academy and the British Library in London. He was the overall winner of the "Excellence in Psychiatry" Award 2017 and was nominated as one of the top four psychiatrists by Hospital Professional News Ireland—Top 100 Professionals in Ireland 2017.

Contents

Preface

The changing face of psychiatry and clinical psychology is mostly illustrated by the hugely increasing prevalence of autism spectrum disorder (ASD) as we increase our understanding and broaden the concept from Leo Kanner's (1943) very narrow concept. The prevalence of ASD was 4/10,000 and is now 1/59, according to the Center for Disease Control in Atlanta, Georgia. Older concepts of autism, that is narrow concepts, have been shown to be completely outdated and unfortunately their use deprives children of ASD diagnosis, with serious consequences for the child, family, and school. A more restricted concept of autism is still contained in instruments, for example, the Autism Diagnostic Interview—Revised and the Autism Diagnostic Observation Scale (ADOS). Parents are still being reduced to tears when they are given a so-called diagnosis of "ADI-negative," and when parents, schools, etc., see clearly that the child has autism. The National Institute for Clinical Excellence Guidelines (2012) specifically point out that there is no precise instrument for the diagnosis of autism and that it is a clinical diagnosis by an expert in autism that is best. According to Baird et al. (2006), about 25/10,000 meet criteria for autism diagnosis based on ADI-ADOS, while the rate of current diagnosis, that is ADS, gives a rate of about 116/10,000. This means that ADI-ADOS is missing over three-quarters of patients who would now be described as having ASD. The rate of expansion of research on ASD is now so rapid that books like this are necessary to bring recent advances together in one place.

This book focuses on the controversies of the diagnosis of ASD with an examination of the putative link between autism, stercobilin, and gastrointestinal disorders. It also focuses on an exploration of scalp acupuncture as a possible treatment. There is also critical examination of autism in the classroom and an investigation into a very unusual phenomenon observed in Uganda called "nodding syndrome."

Michael Fitzgerald
Professor,
Department of Psychiatry,
Trinity College,
Ireland

Chapter 1

Introductory Chapter: Autism Spectrum Disorder - Advances at the End of the Second Decade of the Twenty-First Century

Michael Francis Fitzgerald

1. Introduction

Now, as we move into the third decade of the twenty-first century, it is time to examine some of the current research in autism, for example, microbiome and other research, which is described in this book. Therapies for children with autism continue to be challenging, with no one therapy has been shown to be superior to all other forms of therapy. Indeed, the treatment situation echoes what Lewis Carroll wrote, "*all have won, and all must have prizes*." By that is meant the equivalence of outcome for various therapies for autism. Parents should not engage with therapies promising a cure for autism, however, attractive these promises may be. Nevertheless, a great deal can be achieved with current therapies, including mind reading skills therapy, behaviour therapy, speech and language therapy, occupational therapy and certain medications, if necessary.

2. Diagnosis

Diagnosis is still a problem with some diagnosticians still holding on to outdated concepts like Kanner's autism. Kanner's autism is very real but an extremely rare form of autism, and only a small minority of children meet the criteria for Kanner's autism. Fitzgerald et al. [1] showed that there were different prevalences of diagnosis, depending on which criteria were used:

1. There were 309 with a possible autism diagnosis, of which 285 (85%) met DSM III-R criteria.

2. One hundred forty-four (47%) met ICD-10 criteria.

3. Twenty-four (8%) met Kanner's five criteria.

4. Two-hundred twenty (71%) met Kanner and Eisenberg's two criteria, and nobody met criteria for Asperger's syndrome.

This remains a problem, and it remains to be seen what the final diagnostic criteria for autism spectrum disorder will be. Currently, we use DSM 5 [2]. According to Baird et al. [3], about 25 per 10,000 met criteria for autism diagnosis based on the autism diagnostic interview/autism diagnostic observation scale (ADI-ADOS), while the rate for current diagnosis which would be the autism spectrum disorder gave a rate of about 116 per 10,000. This means ADI-ADOS is missing over three-quarters of patients who would now be described as having an autism spectrum disorder. It is commonly missed by professionals that the diagnosis of autism is a clinical diagnosis by an expert in the diagnosis of autism [4]. Missing autism spectrum disorder has catastrophic effects on the child themselves, the family and school.

Clearly, only those with higher IQ, the standard IQ necessary for university, will move on to a university. One of the most damaging aspects of the school life, which is almost pervasive and long lasting, is bullying. This leads to anxiety, PTSD, and depression in these children, as well as suicidal behaviour.

3. Intervention

It is critical that the quality of training that teachers and classroom assistants have is good. It is almost impossible for those in the classroom to work with children with autism without the clinical autism gestalt. Staff who have this correct sense of the world as seen by a child with autism do extremely good work, become fascinated with the topic and spend the rest of their professional life working with children with autism. Many of the children with autism are the most interesting children a teacher can have the privilege to work with. Many have special talents, and there is a need to build on these special talents and use them in the context of social interaction and building social skills. This will increase the chances of the child living independently and having occupational success later, sometimes which is something that is extremely challenging for persons on the autism spectrum, including those with a high IQ on the autism spectrum. The issues of parent and school relations are very challenging. Because of the nature of autism, both sides can have extreme difficulty seeing things from the others' point of view. Parent/staff meetings will have to be twice as long, when the child has autism because of the difficulties of communication. It is not surprising that staff can feel persecuted and misunderstood because they are speaking on a different level to the parents. The child with autism requires special understanding on the part of the school to understand their difficulties. It is not surprising because of these difficulties that there are often threats of litigation or actual litigation, because of these interpersonal communicational problems.

Of course, it is very easy in these situations for both sides to feel misunderstood. It is sometimes helpful for an outside professional child psychiatrist/child psychologist to be engaged to deal with these difficulties. Children with autism and their autistic friends live in a culture in an autistic culture, and it is necessary for teachers to understand them. Teachers have to be aware of the family's and particularly the child with autism difficulty understanding emotions. It is not rare for more than one member of a family to have autism because it has such a high genetic loading. It is critical that teachers make reference to special autism services when the child is depressed, is very anxious or is making threats of killing themselves, which are far from uncommon. The relationship between the teacher and the outside autism professional will be critical to the child's success in school. Severe depression of psychotic proportions may need to be treated with antidepressants, and attention deficit hyperactivity disorder, which is so often co-morbid with autism, is often missed by child psychologists and child psychiatrists, and this needs to be diagnosed and treated, if the child is to have a successful school outcome. Indeed, untreated children with autism who have also ADHD may be unmanageable in the classroom. They are then excluded, which unfortunately is a very common outcome. There are excellent behavioural strategies for dealing with ADHD, and medications like Ritalin are sometimes necessary as well.

They were drawn to this by previous hypothesis about the opioid excess theory of autism and clinical experience by some of the authors. They observed improvements in autistic behaviour in children on gluten- and casein-free diets. These treatments have been around for over 30 years, have always been controversial, but are now becoming far more central to the treatment and understanding of autism or at least autism subgroups. These theories have not gone away because there was always a kernel of truth in them. I myself have observed a subgroup of patients with autism who have benefitted significantly from gluten- and casein-free diets. Other patients in my experience got no benefit from the diets. The reason is that there is such massive heterogeneity in autism, both at the etiological, clinical presentation and response to treatment level. Someday, we may have biomarkers which will allow us to subtype autism spectrum disorders in a meaningful way. There is no available at this time, but this chapter is working on the possibility of a biomarker. This lack of biomarkers is a central problem in all psychiatry, and we have no biomarkers that can be used clinically in psychiatry, as of now. The scientific study by Ann-Mari Knivsberg and colleagues in 1995 [5] is of critical importance for understanding the relationship between diet and clinical improvement in patients with autism.

Author details

Michael Francis Fitzgerald
Department of Clinical Psychiatry, Trinity College Dublin, Ireland

*Address all correspondence to: profmichaelfitzgerald@gmail.com

References

[1] Fitzgerald M, Matthews P, Birkbeck G, O'Connor J. Irish Families under Stress: Planning for the Future of Autistic Persons. A Prevalence in Psychosocial Study in the Eastern Health Board. Volume 6. Dublin: E.R.H.A; 2000

[2] American Psychiatric Association. DSM 5. Washington, DC: American Psychiatric Association; 2013

[3] Baird G, Simonoff E, Pickles A, Chandler S, Loucas T, Meldrum D, et al. Prevalence of disorders of the autism spectrum in a population cohort of children in South Thames: The special needs and autism project. Lancet. 2006;**368**(9531):210-215

[4] National Institute for Health and Clinical Excellence (NICE). Autism. London: British Psychological Society/ Royal College of Psychiatrists; 2012

[5] Knivsberg AM, Reichelt K, Nodland M, Hoien T. Autistic syndromes and diet: A follow-up study. Scandinavian Journal of Educational Research. 1995;**39**:223-236

Chapter 2

Nodding Syndrome and Autism Spectrum Disorder

David Lagoro Kitara, Denis Anywar Arony and Suzanne Gazda

Abstract

Nodding syndrome (NS) is a devastating childhood neurological disorder seen in clusters in Eastern Africa but of uncertain nosology. It is characterized by repetitive head nodding, atonic seizures, cognitive decline, and school dropout, wasting and stunted growth and it occurs in children subject to internal displacement, food insecurity, and exposure to infectious diseases, contaminated environment and with a number of repetitive behavioral abnormalities. On the other hand autism spectrum disorders (ASD) is a group of behaviorally defined neurodevelopmental disorders with lifelong consequences. They are defined by impairments in communication and social interaction along with restrictive and repetitive behaviors. It is a complex disorder associated with a wide range of disparate and seemingly unrelated factors such as; maternal exposure to various chemical substances, maternal exposure to child abuse, maternal evidence of Diabetes, autoimmune diseases, age of either parents at conception, exposure of infants to various chemical substances, low vitamin D levels of the infant at birth, gender of the infant and a large number of genetic factors. There are a number of similarities in the clinical, biochemical and behavioral findings in children with NS and ASD.

Keywords: nodding syndrome, autism spectrum disorder, Gulu, Uganda

1. Introduction

Nodding syndrome (NS) is a devastating childhood neurological disorder of uncertain nosology [1]. The syndrome is characterized by atonic seizures, head nodding, cognitive decline, muscle weakness, school dropout, thermal dysfunction, internal displacement, food insecurity, wasting, stunted growth, exposures to infectious diseases, contaminated environment and with a number of repetitive behavioral abnormalities [1, 2]. It occurs in clusters in three Eastern African countries (Uganda, Tanzania and South Sudan) and has spatial temporality and clustered in time (during IDP period), space (clustered on either sides of the two main rivers of Aswa and Pager) and person (mainly at 5–15 years of age at onset) particularly in Northern Uganda [3]. The syndrome was first described in 1st scientific meeting organized by the Ugandan Ministry of Health (MOH) and World Health Organization (WHO) in Sheraton, Kampala, Uganda in 2012 [4]. The outcome of the meeting was the agreed WHO epidemiological and surveillance case definition of probable nodding syndrome [5, 6]. It states, "Probable NS cases should meet the following criteria:

- Reported head nodding in a previously normal person who have been observed and recorded by a trained healthcare worker.
- Head nodding is defined as repetitive, involuntary drops of the head to the chest on two or more occasions.
- Age at onset of nodding between 3 and 18 years old.
- Frequency of nodding 5 to 20 per minute.
- Plus at least one of the following criteria:
    - Other neurological abnormalities (cognitive decline, school dropout due to cognitive/behavioral problems, other seizures or neurological abnormalities).
    - Clustering in space or time with similar cases.
    - Triggered by food and/or cold weather.
    - Stunting or wasting.
    - Delayed sexual or physical development.
    - Psychiatric symptoms."

In addition, it has been observed that nodding episodes were stimulated by sights of local food, starvation, exposure to cold weather/temperatures, cold water, stress, physical exercises and there was an association with high anion gap and that most NS began in the internally Displaced Peoples camps (IDPs) or immediately after resettlement into the satellite camps and eventually to their original villages [1–5]. Researchers propose that NS is an emerging neurological disorder in Eastern Africa likely due to factors that were experienced during the IDPs [1, 3–5] and that no new NS cases have been reported since 2012 by the Ugandan Ministry of Health (MOH) and WHO after the IDP camps were disbanded and the affected communities resettled in their villages [1, 3, 5].

Some authors have suggested that nodding syndrome may perhaps be similar to a psychogenic disease (psychogenic illness) in which physical illnesses that are believed to arise from emotional or mental stressors or from psychological or psychiatric disorders may have resulted from the 20 year old civil war that occurred in Northern Uganda. Psychogenic diseases are most commonly applied to illnesses where there is a physical abnormality and other biomarker has not yet been identified as observed in children with NS. Interestingly, the onset of NS perhaps has some similarities to a mass psychogenic illness which involves rapid spread of illness, signs and symptoms affecting a cohesive group originating from a nervous system disturbance involving seizures, loss/reduction of cognitive function with emotional and behavioral abnormalities.

However, findings in NS children contrasts greatly from epidemic hysteria, psychogenic contagion, imitation as perhaps observed among some NS families where two or more children in the same family were affected with the syndrome. Important to note was that all the children that developed NS in the same family did not show evidence of hysterical behavior but physical signs and symptoms that seems to arise from a common experience during the IDPs. Each NS child's presentation vary from each other and perhaps reflecting the spectrum nature of NS occurrence from the most severe to mild form. It was also noted that the course of the NS illness was greatly altered and improved by early initiation of medical intervention on the affected NS child.

The most recent findings through an extensive histoimmunochemistry of brains of deceased nodding syndrome children have revealed that Nodding Syndrome is a tauopathy [7]. This draws more attention to the possibility of diet and environmental exposures of NS children as the likely source of the pathology [3].

Interestingly, all communities where NS occur at epidemic proportion experienced some degree of internal displacement before the onset of NS [2, 3, 5]. In addition, there is a widely held belief among the affected communities in Northern Uganda that NS had possibly originated from contaminated relief food provided during IDPs or exposure to war munitions/chemicals during the protracted 20 year old war in Northern Uganda between the rebel, Lord's Resistance Army (LRA) and the Government of Uganda where 90% of the population in Acholi were displaced into IDPs [8, 9]. Some studies have reported consumption of spoiled relief foods by NS children while in IDPs but there are no mentions of the proportions of NS children that ate it [10–14]. Furthermore, Researchers have extensively investigated cause(s) of NS due to infectious agents but with no single cause that have so far been confirmed [1, 10]. In particular, studies from Northern Uganda have identified high Anion gap metabolic acidosis among NS children compared to their sex and age matched controls [1, 6, 10, 15]. These findings suggested perhaps that NS could be secondary to a metabolic disorder and perhaps a mitochondrial disorder [1, 6, 10, 15]. In addition, researchers observed that nodding episodes were precipitated by sights of local food, starvation, exposure to cold weather/temperatures or cold water, stress, excess physical exercises and there was a statistically significant association with high anion gap [1, 6, 10, 15]. Other researchers suggested that since the IDPs were disbanded, no new NS cases were reported when the affected communities resettled in their villages and feed on their home grown foods [2, 6, 8, 15] an indication that perhaps the factors that led to the onset of the syndrome were removed by moving the communities from the agents that may have been involved in its etiology.

In a recent case control study, researchers found a statistically significant association between NS and biotinidase and acetyl carnitine deficiencies [16]. In addition, other studies had previously observed a deficiency in Vitamin B6 [15] and Vitamin D in NS children [17, 18]. All these findings may suggest perhaps that NS could be secondary to a metabolic disorder and perhaps a mitochondrial disorder may be one of the factors [1, 3–6, 10, 16]. Interestingly, recent data on NS children in a study conducted by a team of researchers from the US funded by National Institute of Health (NIH) suggested an association between NS with cerebrospinal fluid (CSF) VGKC antibodies [19] and serum leiomidin-1 antibody, suggesting a neuroinflammatory cause [20]. All these findings give credence to an emerging neurological disorder which is devastating the lives of many young people in Eastern Africa and that there is no single identifiable marker and that management and prevention strategies have remained elusive.

On the other hand, autism spectrum disorders (ASD) is a group of behaviorally defined neurodevelopmental disorders with lifelong consequences [21]. They are defined by impairments in communication and social interaction along with restrictive and repetitive behaviors [21]. Autism spectrum disorder is now estimated to affect 1 out of 68 individuals in the United States with approximately four times more males than females being affected [22]. Although ASD is behaviorally defined, children with ASD also have many co-occurring medical conditions such as gastrointestinal abnormalities [23], seizures and epilepsy [24], attention deficits [25], anxiety disorders [26] and allergies [27]. It is reported that one of the most significant co morbidities associated with ASD that causes significant disability is epilepsy [28] and a number of studies have suggested that epilepsy affects a high proportion of individuals with ASD [28]. In addition, a number of risk factors for autism can be categorized as risk factors for inflammation or indicators of inflammation [28] which seems to be similar to the factors suggested in the etiology of nodding syndrome.

2. Nodding syndrome and displacement into IDP camps

Several epidemiological studies in Uganda show NS clustered in time (IDP camp period); space (Geographically located on either side of two major rivers (Aswa & Pager) and in person (NS onset is mainly between ages of 5–15 years) [2, 3, 29]. There is an association between life in the IDP camps and onset of NS [2–4, 29]. Historically from 1986 to 2007/2008, Northern Uganda experienced a civil war between the Ugandan Army and rebel groups [2, 30]. Starting in mid-1990s, IDP camps were established in some parts of Northern Uganda with the goal of protecting the population and with an estimated 285,000 people from Kitgum District displaced into IDPs [2, 31, 32]. In the period before displacement into IDPs, there were no reported cases of NS [2]. Similarly in 2001, another community of Aromowanglobo in Awere sub county, Gulu District were moved into IDPs where many of them became dependent on food rations supplied by the relief agencies [3, 33]. IDP camps became associated with malnutrition, social norm breakdown, rising incidence of alcoholism, mental health disorders, suicidal tendencies, increasing prevalence of HIV, Cholera, Hepatitis B & E and other infectious diseases, neglect and waste of the youths [2–4, 29]. The IDPs began to be disbanded in late 2006 when the LRA retreated to South Sudan but during the height of the insurgency in 2002 over 1.5 million people were displaced in the Acholi sub region and thus accounting for over 90% of the population [31, 32]. After 2007, the Government began returning the displaced people into their homes in a phase-wise approach from the main IDPs to satellite camps near their villages [2, 31, 32]. Eventually by 2010, the communities were returned to their original homes in their farmland where the returnees were to settle and rebuild their lives [2–4, 31, 32].

In 2009, the Ugandan Ministry of Health (MOH) identified NS in communities in Northern Uganda and later on established NS screening and rehabilitation centers in 2012 where NS children were treated with anticonvulsants, multivitamins and nutritional supplements [3, 5, 6, 10, 19, 29]. The consistency of supplies and rehabilitation processes faced challenges including irregular supply of anticonvulsants and food for NS children and the vulnerable families [2, 8, 9, 31, 32]. In the same period, there was an apparent relationship between the peaks of NS cases in Kitgum District and earlier peak influxes of households into IDPs [2] which was similarly observed in Awere Sub County in Gulu district [3]. Important to note was that the 1997 peak influx of IDPs in Kitgum District was followed 7 years later by an elevated number of new NS cases in 2004 (2003–2005) and similarly in the 2003 large influx of households had a larger peak in new NS cases 5 years later in 2008 [2]. This was similarly observed in Awere in Gulu where the 2001–2002 influxes were followed with increased incidences of NS, 7 years later in 2008–2009 [3]. The peaks of reported NS onset correlated with peaks of household displacement and food insecurity, where residents were heavily dependent on food aid from relief agencies [2, 3, 29, 31–34]. The IDP camps were exceptionally poor, insecure, unsanitary, with overcrowding, violence, food insecurity and squalid, and morbidity and mortality rates were high [2, 35].

In 2005, a Government survey of Kitgum district estimated an IDP population of 310,111 persons; 21% of whom were children under 5 years [2]. At the time of the survey, over 66% of children were reported to have been ill sometime in the previous 2 weeks and the crude mortality rates were reported to be 2 deaths per 10,000 per day and double that rate for children under the age of 5 years [2, 29, 35]. In addition, the top self-reported causes of death in IDPs were malaria/fever (34.7%), AIDS (15.1%) and violence (10.5%) [2] and water was obtained from protected sources but water intake was low and the waiting time was high and the infant feeding practices were poor [2]. It is reported that for children under the age of 5 years, the traditional disease concept of "Two Lango" or "Gin pa Omiru" which was a combination of oral thrush, malnutrition and diarrhea was the second most commonly reported causes of death [2, 34]. These findings were thorough analysis of the events in all IDPs across the Acholi and Lango sub regions where NS occurred at epidemic proportions.

3. Epidemiological, environmental and dietary findings on nodding syndrome children

Studies show that NS in Awere, Gulu district, Northern Uganda was first noted in 2002 which corresponded with 1 year stay in IDPs [3]. The month of peak incidence of NS onset was April and October [3]. These peaks corresponded fairly with the peaks of monthly average rainfall for 1st and 2nd rainy seasons [3] and related to scarcity of food as observed by Landis et al. [2]. The factors around the syndrome onset could have perhaps been in IDPs since all NS children were in IDPs before onset of nodding [2, 3, 29]. The other reason could perhaps be that NS children who were born before IDPs, had developed NS earlier except, the condition was not detected or overtly manifested but that the IDP camp conditions precipitated its overt manifestation perhaps coupled with other stressor factors such as *Onchocerca Volvulus* (*OV*) infection; malnutrition, war trauma and febrile illnesses [1–5, 29]. In addition, most NS children were in 1st, 2nd and 3rd birth orders in descending orders respectively [3, 5] and all of them experienced IDP life which peaked at 5 years of IDP stay [3]. Additionally, most NS children have other siblings with NS and its occurrence in siblings mirrored NS children's birth orders [3]. This finding, perhaps point towards a possibility of an acquired disease which was overtly manifested possibly as a result of family/household factors such as; poor storage of food leading to contamination and/or infection with *OV* or stress which made the syndrome perhaps manifestly overt on exposure to these factors [3, 5]. Perhaps the perfect examples of such could be seen in deficiencies of metabolites in acquired diseases whose disease occurrence becomes overtly expressed in circumstances of stress [36]. That could perhaps explain why there are no new NS cases since 2012 when the communities were resettled in their villages and feed on their own home grown foods [3, 19, 29, 37].

In general, the information provided by parents of NS children show that NS children were all reported to have been born normal and that the developmental milestones were normal until NS began [1, 3, 5, 29, 37, 38]. Before onset of nodding, food listed in [3, 5] were the supplementary and weaning foods that were supplied by relief agencies and eaten by the IDPs residents including NS children [31]. The quantity and duration of these food ration eaten by each NS child could however, not be determined but report on it was provided by the World Food Program (WFP) [31, 32].

Interestingly in 2012 when some NS children were examined before admission to the Hope for HumaNs (HfH) centre for NS rehabilitation, they were diagnosed mostly with Severe Acute Malnutrition (SAM) and a few with Moderate Acute Malnutrition (MAM) respectively on the basis of their z-scores [38]. Upon enrolment for a multidisciplinary and syndromic treatment with anticonvulsants, multivitamins, local food supplements, and psychosocial support; their health conditions greatly improved, seizure frequency reduced, mental health status improved, cognitive impairment improved, they gained weight and height and by 2014 when the author re-assessed these NS children in a longitudinal study, most of them had improved and categorized as MAM and healthy nutritionally [5, 29, 38, 39]. This observation was perhaps due to good feeding program at the HfH centre and adequate rehabilitation processes accorded to NS children. However, much as they had improved and some had returned to school, none of them could be declared cured because they still experienced sporadic episodes of nodding, emotional and perceptual disturbances and some cognitive impairment [5, 10, 29, 38, 39].

4. Biotinidase and acetyl carnitine deficiency, nodding syndrome and metabolic disorder

In one of the pilot studies conducted on NS children in Northern Uganda, it was observed that most NS children demonstrated a deficiency of biotinidase enzyme activity ranging from 0 to 100% [16]. The average percentage deficiency was 78% (78 SD $\pm$ 13.362), an indication that this enzymatic deficiency was a spectrum which varied considerably from one NS child to another depending on the percentage deficiency of biotinidase activity [40–43] just like the severity and clinical presentations of NS varied from one child to another [5]. Biotinidase deficiency has commonly been classified as partial or profound deficiency whereby the clinical presentations and occurrence depended on the percentage deficiency and the presence of stressor factors [40–43]. It is reported that partial biotinidase deficiency is a milder form of this condition in which without treatment with biotin, the affected child may experience hypotonia, skin rashes and hair loss, but these problems may appear only during illness, infections, or other times of stress [40–43]. These authors suggest that NS occurs as a spectrum similarly to biotinidase deficiency and that for NS children that had partial biotinidase deficiency, they experienced severe stress (Malnutrition, psychological stress and *OV* infection) that resulted into the overt presentation of NS [16]. The stressors in this case could have perhaps been the IDP camp life, where there was inadequate food for consumption (with resultant malnutrition) [31, 32, 35] or infection with *Onchocerca volvulus* which afflicted nearly 80% of NS children or psychological stress [1, 4, 17]. Other stressors could have been severe illnesses such as malaria, meningitis, cholera and others which were common in the IDP camps and affected a large number of IDP residents [2, 35, 44]. On the other hand profound biotinidase deficiency is a more severe and can cause seizures, weak muscle tone (hypotonia), breathing problems, hearing and vision loss, problems with movement and balance (ataxia), skin rashes, hair loss (alopecia) and fungal infection particularly candidiasis [40–43]. The affected children with biotinidase deficiency also have delayed development miles stones [40–43]. Most of these symptoms and signs were similarly observed in NS children in Northern Uganda.

The clinical presentations of NS children examined in 2012 and repeated in 2014 as part of a longitudinal study are similar to the clinical presentations of biotinidase deficiency [39]. However, hearing and vision loss which are typically seen in profound biotinidase deficiency were not observed in 2014 perhaps due to 2 years of rehabilitation where it is suspected that the symptoms and signs which were akin to profound biotinidase activity deficiency could not all be observed [39]. It is important to note that biotinidase functions by recycling the vitamin biotin which is also known as vitamin B7 and it is bound to amino groups of lysine residues of apoenzymes [41–43, 45]. If levels of serum biotinidase are low then biotin cannot be broken down and released from proteins into the diet [41–43, 45]. In addition, biotin serves as a coenzyme for four carboxylases enzymes; propionyl-CoA carboylases & β-methyl crotonyl-CoA carboxylases, which are important in protein catabolism; pyruvate carboxylases, which are essential for gluconeogenesis and acetyl CoA carboxylases, which are involved in the first step in fatty acid synthesis [42, 45]. Similarly, the majority of the NS children had deficiency of the acetyl carnitine, a metabolite responsible for the transfer of short chain fatty acids into the mitochondrium for metabolism and this perhaps represented the view that at the time of stress, NS children were unable to utilize the short chain fatty acids and perhaps with the resultant observed clinical features. Similarly, a previous study had noted a near significant association between NS and pyridoxine deficiency (Bunga's study ($p = 0.06$)) [11].This finding was very important as seizures are normally associated with abnormal pyridoxine metabolism [11].

In the same study, the levels of serum urate were overall unremarkable, demonstrating that NS wasn't perhaps associated with abnormalities involving purine or pyrimidine metabolism [16]. The urate/creatinine ratio levels were lower than normal range, suggesting that NS was not probably associated with rhabdomyolysis [16]. In addition, it was previously observed by another author that NS was associated with vitamin D deficiency in which 7 out of 8 NS cases had reported vitamin D deficiency [17]. Furthermore, findings from other studies indicate that the levels of organic acid in urine were generally high and this was consistent with other findings of high anion gap metabolic acidosis seen in NS patients in a case control study [1]; case series [17]; case reports [10, 15] and clinical studies [39].

Therefore, NS in South Sudan & Northern Uganda represents an emerging neurological disorder where investigations searching for potential environmental toxins have not yet been fully conducted [4, 29, 46]. It is reported that thousands of pesticides, solvents and other industrial chemicals have not been tested for neurodevelopmental toxicity in the community where NS occurs at epidemic proportions [46]. Historically, it has taken several decades of scrutiny to confirm developmental neurotoxicity secondary to industrial chemicals following initial clinical diagnosis of poisoning [47]. In South Sudan in 2011, CDC study collected urine and blood and did analysis for heavy metals; however the preliminary analysis of blood and urine results remains unpublished [48]. Bunga's (2011) Sudanese unpublished study mentioned in Dowell et al.'s study, found no abnormality detected in the urine for mercury, thiocyanate and arsenic [11]. Foltz et al., tested serum for copper and urine for homocysteine & thiocyanate levels [49]; Sevjar et al. reported to have had an unremarkable toxin analysis (data not shown) [50]. The vast majority of investigations into possible neurotoxic causes to NS children came from information regarding diet, collected via questionnaires from NS caregivers [14, 18, 46, 51–54]. There have been associations that have been demonstrated between eating red sorghum and NS in a South Sudan study [46]. It has also been further reported that there is an unidentified associated with mycotoxins which was suggested as a likely putative agent [4, 29, 46]. Interestingly to date, there is no published laboratory microbiological or neurotoxicological analysis of food that was eaten in the IDPs camps to confirm these hypotheses. Further to this, NS in South Sudan and Northern Uganda is suspected to be caused by a chemical neurotoxin from war munitions used during the civil wars [8, 9, 46]. However, there are no published studies investigating quantifiable war munitions and/or chemicals as possible cause(s), despite several case control studies demonstrating a positive association with exposure to war munitions and gun raids [11, 46, 49]. However, a recent case series in Northern Uganda found that all NS children had been exposed to either severe war-related psychological and physical trauma and that most of those interviewed in an observational study laid blame on war munitions/chemicals [8, 55]. These findings showed that the environmental exposures of the affected communities were reported although not proven but still forms a basis for hypothesis that it could be a factor that could not be ignored in the epidemiology of NS in Northern and South Sudan.

5. Experience of treatment and rehabilitation of children with nodding syndrome

The treatment and rehabilitation responses of NS children in Northern Uganda by Hope for HumaNs (HfH) has registered positive outcome with improved mid upper arm circumference (MUAC), height, weight and hematological indices [39]. The comprehensive rehabilitation approach (correcting protein-energy using MAMA nutritional food supplements and vitamin-related malnutrition, deworming, oral fungicide, anti-seizure medications (sodium valproate with/or without Carbamazepine); close monitoring; tailored dosing and adjustments; special needs education program; counseling) pioneered by HfH at Odek rehabilitation centre has proven clinically transformative (steady growth, improved emotional and marked seizure reduction status—though greater among males than females for unknown reasons) [3, 4, 38]. It was still noted though that cognitive, behavioral problems and social difficulties still confronted these NS children even 9 months after rehabilitation at the HfH centre [39].

6. Nodding syndrome (NS), biotinidase and acetyl carnitine deficiency and autism spectrum disorder (ASD)

Although autism spectrum disorder (ASD) was originally thought to be a static, inheritable neurodevelopmental disorder, its understanding is currently undergoing a major shift [45]. It is now emerging as a dynamic system of metabolic and immune anomalies involving many organ systems, including the brain and environmental exposures [45, 56]. The initial detailed observation and inquiry on patients with ASD and related conditions, the histories of their caregivers and families have been providing important information [45]. To date, it is not yet clear how gastrointestinal (GI) factors are related to ASD [45, 56] however, many patients with ASD have a history of previous antibiotic exposure or hospitalization, GI symptoms, abnormal food cravings and unique intestinal bacterial populations, which have been proposed to relate to variable symptom severity [45, 57]. An author recently recommended that new approaches would be required to examine the diverse symptoms and co morbidities of this growing family of neurodevelopmental disorders known as autism spectrum disorder [45]. It is reported that neurochemical changes which is consistent and predictive with findings in ASD patients, including neuroinflammation, increased oxidative stress, mitochondrial dysfunction, glutathione depletion and altered phospholipids/acylcarnitine profiles, have been observed [45, 57]. In addition, propionic acid have been reported to have bioactive effects on; neurotransmitter systems; intracellular acidification and calcium release; fatty acid metabolism; gap junction gating; immune function and alteration of gene expression that warrant further exploration [45]. Furthermore, other authors have proposed that traditional scientific experimentation was required to verify the hypothesis that enteric short-chain fatty acids may be a potential environmental trigger in some forms of ASD [45, 56, 58]. Interestingly, the collaborative developments in systems biology particularly examining the role of microbiome and its effects on host metabolism, immune and mitochondrial function and gene expression, is reported to hold a great promise in investigation on ASD [23, 45, 58–61]. It is further suggested that the microbiome produces an array of bioactive metabolic products capable of entering systemic circulation [23, 45, 61]. Other authors have suggested that enteric microbiome and its metabolic products were dynamic and could be altered throughout an individual's life cycle, particularly during the first 18 months of life [57–60, 62]. In addition, it was reported that the metabolic products from the GI tract microbiome could have profound and dynamic effects on host metabolism, immune functions and gene expressions which happens in many organ systems including the CNS [58]. Furthermore, other authors recommended that it was important to consider the effects of infant formula versus breastfeeding, a high-calorie Western diet and exposure to antibiotics and disinfectants in human beings, animals and plants on the alteration of the human microbiome and its metabolites [45, 54, 56, 63, 64]. These should be considered a possible source of environmental triggers of many diseases of increasing incidence including ASD [45]. This was particularly evident from human populations who migrated to Western societies, such as the Somalis in the diaspora, who appeared to have a much higher incidence of ASD than it existed in their country of origin [45, 65].

Furthermore, there are examples of this experience in biology to show that it may be possible that GI biome could alter the behaviors of animals [45, 66–68]. Examples; Rabies and *Bornavirus* infect the CNS in animals and induce aggression that spreads the virus in the saliva from one animal to another through biting behaviors [45]; Cordyceps (*Ophiocordyceps unilateralis*) is a fungal infection that affects the behavior of ants, causing them to climb to the top of plants before they die [45]. The resulting fruiting bodies of the fungus then sprout out of the dead insect to spread spores [45]; in addition, *Toxoplasmosis* causes rodents to act without an appropriate fear response, leading to transmission of the infectious agent through cats via predation and ultimately on to humans [45]; Furthermore, Mundane acts such as sneezing with a common cold or increased gastric motility leading to nausea and vomiting in viral gastroenteritis are said to be in the best interest of spreading the infectious agent [45]. The researcher then ponders whether similar things that happen such as carbohydrate craving, diarrhea and fecal smearing in ASD helps to feed and spread bacteria? [45]. It was observed that families of ASD children just like NS children often become more alienated when they are told about their children's regression condition and that there was not much that could be done [45] and they were often encouraged to use medications to partially reduce aggressive behavior and to wait for their turn for the under-funded behavioral intervention programs that take years to begin and years to complete [45, 56]. The strain and stress of dealing with these children can destroy families and end productive careers, leading desperate and vulnerable parents to turn to unproven controversial treatments that can be costly, potentially dangerous and without confirmed effectiveness [45]. This has been observed in parents of children with NS who have in their helplessness resorted to the use of traditional medicines including and not limited to the use of crashed roots, traditional medicines, witchcrafts, prayers, visits to shrines and animal sacrifices as remedies for the treatment of this syndrome [10, 15, 46, 50]. In addition, there are new interesting issues to learn about some observations of bizarre food cravings, GI symptoms, epilepsy, infectious processes and metabolic disturbances in children affected with ASD [45, 68–70] just like for the NS children. However, there were reports that some ASD children appeared to improve, either spontaneously, after certain broad spectrum antibiotics, or possibly by altering their diet [45]. This particular scenario has been observed in NS children at the HfH rehabilitation centre in which NS children whose feeding pattern (using a locally prepare MAMA food supplement) and symptomatic treatment have made them improve physically but still confronted with cognitive, emotional and perceptual difficulties [3, 4, 38, 39]. A researcher wonders whether there might be a common digestive system link to these findings even if current understanding in conventional western medicine could do little for these ASD and NS children. The mitochondrial disorders observed in ASD—studied extensively by Dan Rossignol, Rossignol Medical Center, Irvine, California, and Richard Frye, University of Arkansas, appeared to occur largely through environmental and not inherited means [45, 71, 72]. It is reported that these disorders observed might be caused by or at least worsened by enteric short-chain fatty acids including propionic acid from GI tract bacteria [45, 57, 71, 72]. This is similarly a suggestion being advanced on NS children seen in Northern Uganda and South Sudan because first, they were made to feed on food provided by the relief agencies which were not their usual diet during IDPs period (plumpy nuts, powdered milk, soya beans, red sorghum, cooking oil which were sometimes of uncertain composition, rice, yellow posho and other food substances that were made available to them) [3]. Secondly, there have been consistent observation in case control studies, case series, case reports and clinical and biochemical studies that NS children do have high anion gap metabolic acidosis with depleted bicarbonate levels and one author proposed that the cause of this syndrome may perhaps be due to mitochondrial disorders, a factor which may be common to ASD and NS [1, 2, 10, 15, 50]. The cooking oil supplied and consumed by the IDP residents provided by the relief agencies were not common to their GI microbiome but may have perhaps been those of short chain fatty acids [1–3, 5].

Furthermore, the reported collaborative work of Dr. Frye, who reviewed his ASD patient population and found a large subset with the lipid (acylcarnitine) and biochemical (citric acid, glutathione) findings predicted by the propionic rodent model was another breakthrough in the advancement of science of ASD [45, 71–74]. His finding in June 2012, that there was an absence of genetic abnormalities to explain these changes in ASD, suggesting that the biochemical findings stemmed from environmental factors and were not inherited [45, 73, 74]. These similar findings were observed in NS children in Northern Uganda where there have been observed acetyl carnitine and biotinidase deficiency in a pilot study conducted on NS children undergoing rehabilitation at the HfH centre [5].

In addition, a recently work with Bistra Nankova, from New York Medical College, found that short chain fatty acids, including propionic acid are histone deacetylase inhibitors and thus were switchers for genes particularly those involved in the metabolism of catecholamines and was important in anxiety, arousal, movement disorders, aggression and cravings [45]. This brings to mind a thought that potentially bacteria can control and tinker with our metabolisms and even human genes [45]. Additionally, some researchers now argue that these bacteria, through natural selection, may be controlling or modulating our behavior and they may serve the host well until environmental factors such as the Western diet or overuse of antibiotics reset the microbiome to produce alterations of this behavior—the obsessions, perseverations, food fixations and tics but also at times enhanced memory associated with ASD [45, 75–80].

The author argued that it was important to note that propionic acid affects multiple systems at different developmental periods in a complex manner and that the evidence of increased propionic acid or other short-chain enteric fatty acids involved in the pathophysiology of ASD, although compelling, was still circumstantial [45, 77–79]. These researchers further reported that propionic and related short-chain fatty acids could elicit behaviors that are anxiety-like, perseverative, repetitive, ritualistic and antisocial [80–84]. These behaviors were reported to be common to many other neuropsychiatric conditions (obsessive compulsive, mood, anxiety, attention deficit/hyperactive and eating disorders, irritable bowel syndrome, and schizophrenia) where infectious agents have been proposed [45, 81, 84]. In addition, the researchers argued that there was a growing incidence of ASD and ASD-related conditions, coupled with the observed alterations in the human microbiome secondary to dietary, medical and agricultural factors and their potential effects on human and animal behavior should be examined further [45, 58, 60, 81, 85, 86]. Professor Jared Diamond contended in his book *Guns, Germs, and Steel* that the impact of human migration and urbanization, domestication of plants and animals and resultant human diseases shaping cultures was not trivial [87]. He further stated that, it was not so far-fetched to say that Western society has altered human microbial populations, which in turn may be altering human behavior and culture [87]. The similarities in the clinical presentations and the biochemical findings in children with NS and ASD draws the attention of these researchers to perhaps an understanding that NS may perhaps be a condition akin to autism spectrum disorder (ASD); a disease spectrum that is not well understood but continues to ravage the lives of many young people and families in developing and developed world akin to the experience of NS in the East Africa. Nodding syndrome were seen only in children who were born normal, lived in the IDP camps, were from poor families, all ate food ration from relief agencies foreign to their GIT and that all the children who developed NS were IDP resident at some stage in their lives [2–5]. The relief agencies distributed various forms of cereals (Plumpy nuts, Beans, soya, red sorghum, yellow posho, and maize) and cooking oil which were perhaps foreign to their GI microbiome of the affected communities and the communities ate them, they provided cooking oil whose constituents were foreign to the population and they consumed them [2, 3, 33, 34]. In addition, NS children have been found to have deficiency of Vitamin B6, Vitamin D, Acetyl carnitine and biotinidase [5]. These factors point to the changes in the diet of the children and adults in these communities where NS occurs at epidemic proportions during and after the war and/or IDPs camp life which may have perhaps been partly responsible for the syndrome that we have been investigating without finding the cause [2, 3, 5]. Important to note was that the Ugandan Ministry of Health and World Health organization have since 2012 reported no new cases of NS in Northern Uganda since the IDP camps were disbanded and communities returned to their farmland and feed on their locally grown foods [2–5]. Therefore autism spectrum disorder, nodding syndrome, biotinidase and acetyl carnitine deficiency [1–3, 5, 88] may be conditions that share many things in common and this may be the right moment to think of considering them as similar/common entities.

7. Conclusion

Nodding syndrome (NS) is a childhood neurological disorder that occurs in clusters in Eastern Africa and of uncertain nosology. However, studies have demonstrated biotinidase and acetyl carnitine deficiency, Vitamin B6 deficiency, high anion gap metabolic acidosis and Vitamin D deficiency. In addition, NS children experienced internal displacement, fed on IDP diets which were mainly foreign to their GI microbiome and other environmental exposures, exposure to wartime situations and infectious diseases at childhood. Rehabilitated of NS children using home grown food supplement (MAMA supplement plus other symptomatic remedies), their conditions improved tremendously and some have returned to school although there is no clear evidence that they have been completely cured. Furthermore, there are no new cases of NS as reported by the Ugandan Ministry of Health (MOH) and World Health Organization (WHO) since 2012 when the IDP camps were disbanded and communities resettled in their own communities and feed on their own home grown foods. Although these findings are inconclusive at this stage, perhaps NS observed in this region may be akin to autism spectrum disorder (ASD).

Acknowledgements

The authors acknowledge the support of Hope for HumaNs (HfH), an NGO which contributed tremendously towards the rehabilitation of NS children for over 5 years. Gulu University, an academic institution which has provided logistical and administrative support to the authors for this book chapter.

Conflict of interest

All authors declare no conflict of interest.

Author details

David Lagoro Kitara[1*], Denis Anywar Arony[2] and Suzanne Gazda[3]

1 Department of Surgery, Faculty of Medicine, Gulu University, Gulu, Uganda

2 Department of Biochemistry, Faculty of Medicine, Gulu University, Gulu, Uganda

3 Neurological Clinic, San Antonio, Texas, United States

*Address all correspondence to: klagoro@gmail.com

References

[1] Kitara DL, Anywar AD, Mwaka AD, Uwonda G, Abwang B, Kigonya E. Nodding syndrome in northern Uganda: A probable metabolic disorder. British Journal of Medical and Health Research. 2013;**3**(4):2054-2068

[2] Landis JL, Palmer VS, Spencer PS. Nodding syndrome in Kitgum District, Uganda: Association with conflict and internal displacement. British Medical Journal Open. 2014;**4**:e006195. DOI: 10.1136/bmjopen-2014-006195

[3] Anywar AD, Angwech C, Makumbi EF, Suzanne G, Kitara DL. Is there a line between internal displacement; environmental and dietary factors in the onset of nodding syndrome in northern Uganda? A clinical observational study design. World Journal of Pharmaceutical and Medical Research. 2017;**3**(9):34-48

[4] Spencer PS, Kitara DL, Gazda SK, Winkler AS. Nodding syndrome 2015: International Conference Report and Gulu Accord. eNeurologicalSci. 2015; **3**(2016):80-83

[5] Anywar AD, Suzanne G, Kitara DL. Could nodding syndrome in northern Uganda be a form of autism spectrum disorder? An observational study design. The Pan African Medical Journal. 2018; **30**:115. DOI: 10.11604/pamj.2018.30.115.13634

[6] Kitara DL, Jason O, Mwaka AD. Nodding syndrome in Uganda—A disease cluster: An epidemiological dilemma. Pacific Journal of Medical Sciences. 2013;**11**(1):21-33

[7] Pollanen MS, Onzivua S, Robertson J, McKeever PM, Wong A, Kitara DL. Nodding syndrome in Uganda is a tauopathy. Acta Neuropathologica. DOI: 10.1007/s00401-018-1909-9

[8] Mitchell KB, Kornfeld J, Adiama J. Nodding syndrome in northern Uganda: Overview and community perspectives. Epilepsy & Behavior. 2013;**26**(1):22-24

[9] Kitara DL, Amone C. Perception of the population in northern Uganda to nodding syndrome. Journal of Medicine and Medical Sciences. 2012;**3**(7): 464-470

[10] Kitara DL, Mwaka AD, Wabinga HR, Bwangamoi PO. Pyomyositis in nodding syndrome (NS) patient: A case report. The Pan African Medical Journal. 2013;**16**:65. DOI: 10.11604/pamj.2013.16.65.2403

[11] Dowell SF, Sejvar JJ, Riek L, Vandemaele KA, Lamunu M, Kuesel AC, et al. Nodding syndrome. Emerging Infectious Diseases. 2013;**19**(9): 1374-1384

[12] Tumwine JK, Vandemaele K, Chungong S, Richer M, Anker M, Ayana Y. Clinical and epidemiologic characteristics of nodding syndrome in Mundri County, South Sudan. African Health Sciences. 2012;**12**(3):242-248

[13] Nyungura JL, Akim T, Lako A. Investigation into nodding syndrome in Witto Payam, Western Equatoria state. Southern Sudan Medical Journal. 2010; **4**:3-6

[14] Winkler AS, Friedrich K, König R, Meindl M, Helbok R, Unterberger I, et al. The head nodding syndrome—Clinical classification and possible causes. Epilepsia. 2008;**49**(12): 2008-2015

[15] Kitara DL, Gazda S, Eger A, Okot A, Angwech C, Valerie SP, et al. Nodding episodes and high anion gap in a 13 year old nodding syndrome child. A case report. British Journal of Medicine and Medical Research. 2014;**6**(8):851-858

[16] Anywar DA, Galloway P, Angwech C, Makumbi EF, Kitara DL. Metabolic analyses of nodding syndrome in Uganda: A pilot study is a biotinidase and acetyl carnitine deficiency; a metabolic disorder. An observational study design. World Journal of Pharmaceutical and Medical Research. 2018;**4**(1):160-174

[17] Kitara DL, Mwaka AD, Kigonya E. High anion gap metabolic acidosis in children with nodding syndrome in northern Uganda. A case series. British Journal of Medicine and Medical Research. 2014;**4**(6):1301-1314

[18] Piloya-Were T, Odongkara-Mpora B, Namusoke H, Idro R. Physical growth, puberty and hormones in adolescents with nodding syndrome; a pilot study. BMC Research Notes. 2014; 7:858

[19] Idro R, Opar B, Wamala J, Abbo C, Onzivua S, Mwaka DA, et al. Is nodding syndrome an *Onchocerca volvulus*-induced neuroinflammatory disorder? Uganda's story of research in understanding the disease. International Journal of Infectious Diseases. 2016;**45**: 112-117

[20] Johnson TP, Tyagi R, Lee PR, Lee MH, Johnson KR, Kowalak J. Nodding syndrome may be an autoimmune reaction to the parasitic worm *Onchocerca volvul*us. Science Translational Medicine. 2017;**9**(377): eaaf6953

[21] Keil A, Daniels JL, Forssen U. Parental autoimmune diseases associated with autism spectrum disorders in offspring. Epidemiology. 2010;**21**:805-808

[22] Tanne JH. Maternal obesity and diabetes are linked to children's autism and similar disorders. BMJ. 2012;**344**: e2768

[23] Atladottir HO, Henriksen TB, Schendel DE. Autism after infection, febrile episodes, and antibiotic use during pregnancy: An exploratory study. Pediatrics. 2012;**130**:e1447-e1454

[24] Parker W, Perkins SE, Harker M. A prescription for clinical immunology: The pills are available and ready for testing. Current Medical Research and Opinion. 2012;**28**:1193-1202

[25] Brenner SL, Jones JP, Rutanen-Whaley RH. Evolutionary mismatch and chronic psychological stress. Journal of Evolutionary Medicine. 2015;**3**:235885

[26] Holick MF. Vitamin D deficiency. The New England Journal of Medicine. 2007;**357**:266-281

[27] Bilbo SD, Wray GA, Perkins SE, Sarah EP. Reconstitution of the human biome as the most reasonable solution for epidemics of allergic and autoimmune diseases. Medical Hypotheses. 2011;**77**(4):494-504. DOI: 10.1016/j.mehy.2011.06.019

[28] Parker W, Chi Dang H, Staci B, Zoie EH, Lauren G, Rasika R, et al. The role of oxidative stress, inflammation and acetaminophen exposure from birth to early childhood in the induction of autism. The Journal of International Medical Research. 2017;**45**(2):407-438

[29] Spencer PS, Mazumder R, Valerie SP, Lasarev MR, Stadnik RC, King P, et al. Other members of the Oregon-Uganda nodding syndrome research team: Environmental, dietary and case-control study of nodding syndrome in Uganda: A post-measles brain disorder triggered by malnutrition? Journal of the Neurological Sciences. 2016;**369**: 191-203

[30] Otunnu O. Causes and Consequences of the War in Acholiland. Available from: http://home.cc.uma

nitoba.ca/~chaser/readings/Armed%20conflict%20and%20Uganda/Northern%20Uganda%20Causes%20and%20consequences%20of%20the%20war%20in%20Acholiland.htm [Accessed: January 5, 2016]

[31] World Food Program. Emergency Food Security Assessment of IDP Camps in Gulu, Kitgum, Kira and Pader Districts, March–May 2005. September 2005. Available from: http://documents.wfp.org/stellent/groups/public/documents/ena/wfp079422.pdf [Accessed: July 10, 2014]

[32] World Food Program. Food Security Assessment of IDP Camps in Gulu, Kitgum, and Pader Districts, October 2006. Final Report. January 2007. Available from: http://documents.wfp.org/stellent/groups/public/documents/ena/wfp120444.pdf [Accessed: July 10, 2014]

[33] Suzanne G, Kitara DL. Could nodding syndrome (NS) in northern Uganda be part of the microbiota-gut-brain axis syndrome? The Pan African Medical Journal. 2018;**31**:152. DOI: 10.11604/pamj.2018.31.152.14142

[34] Anon. Abducted and abused: Renewed conflict in northern Uganda. Human Rights Watch. 2003;**15**:12A. Available from: http://www.hrw.org/sites/default/files/reports/uganda0703.pdf [Accessed: July 2014]

[35] Bozzoli C, Brzzo T. Child mortality and camp decongestion in post-war Uganda. Microcon Research Working Paper 24, Brighton, May 2010. Available from: http://www.microconflict.eu/publications/RWP24_CB_TB.pdf [Accessed: July 10, 2014]

[36] Germaine LD. Biotinidase deficiency clinical presentations. In: Drugs and Diseases. Paediatrics: Genetics and Metabolic Diseases. 2016

[37] Valdes R, Suits A, Valerie P, Okot C, Gazda S, Moka L, et al. A real-time medical cartography of epidemic disease (nodding syndrome) using village-based lay mHealth reporters. PLoS Neglected Tropical Diseases. 2018 (PNTD-D-18-00399R1)- [EMID:98b7bcb993d3641d]

[38] Anywar DA, Suzanne G, Kitara DL. Treatment and rehabilitation outcomes of children affected with nodding syndrome in northern Uganda: A descriptive case series. The Pan African Medical Journal. 2018;**29**:228. DOI: 10.11604/pamj.2018.29.228.13627

[39] Kitara DL, Suzanne G. Nodding syndrome in northern Uganda; treatment and rehabilitation outcomes: A longitudinal study design. World Journal of Pharmaceutical Research. 2017;**6**(14):150-169

[40] Hannigan S. Inherited Metabolic Conditions. A Guide to 100 Conditions. Radcliffe Publishing Ltd; 2007

[41] Wolf B. Biotinidase deficiency: "If you have to have an inherited metabolic disease, this is the one to have". Genetics in Medicine. 2012;**14**:565-575

[42] Wolf B. Clinical issues and frequent questions about biotinidase deficiency. Molecular Genetics and Metabolism. 2010;**100**(1):6-13. DOI: 10.1016/j.ymgme.2010.01.003

[43] Wolf B. The neurology of biotinidase deficiency. Molecular Genetics and Metabolism. 2011;**104**(1–2):27-34

[44] Accorsi S, Fabiani M, Nattabi B, Corrado B, Iriso R, Ayella EO, et al. The disease profile of poverty: Morbidity and mortality in northern Uganda in the context of war, population displacement and HIV/AIDS. Transactions of the

Royal Society of Tropical Medicine and Hygiene;**99**(3):226-233

[45] MacFabe D. Autism: Metabolism, mitochondria, and the microbiome. Global Advances in Health and Medicine. 2013;**2**(6):52-66

[46] Spencer PS, Vandemaele K, Richer M, Palmer VS, Chungong S, Anker M, et al. Nodding syndrome in Mundri County, South Sudan: Environmental, nutritional, and infectious factors. African Health Sciences. 2013;**13**(2): 183-204

[47] Grandjean P, Landrigan PJ. Neurobehavioural effects of developmental toxicology. The Lancet Neurology. 2014; **13**(3):330-338

[48] Centers for Disease Control and Prevention (CDC). Nodding syndrome—South Sudan, 2011. Morbidity and Mortality Weekly Report. 2012;**61**(3):52-54

[49] Foltz JL, Makumbi I, Sejvar JJ, Malimbo M, Ndyomugyenyi R, Atai-Omoruto AD, et al. An epidemiologic investigation of potential risk factors for nodding syndrome in Kitgum District, Uganda. PLoS One. 2013;**18**(8):6, e66419

[50] Sejvar JJ, Kakooza AM, Foltz JL, Makumbi I, Atai-Omoruto AD, Malimbo M, et al. Clinical, neurological, and electrophysiological features of nodding syndrome in Kitgum, Uganda: An observational case series. Lancet Neurology. 2013;**12**(2):166-174

[51] Buchmann K. 'You sit in fear': Understanding perceptions of nodding syndrome in post-conflict northern Uganda. Global Health Action. 2014; **21**(7):25069

[52] Andreas SW, Katrin F, Mitchel M. Clinical characteristics of people with head nodding in southern Tanzania. Tropical Doctor. 2010;**10**(3):173-175

[53] Winkler AS, Friedrich K, Velicheti S, Dharsee J, König R, Nassri A, et al. MRI findings in people with epilepsy and nodding syndrome in an area endemic for onchocerciasis: An observational study. African Health Sciences. 2013;**13**(2):529-540

[54] Winkler AS, Wallner B, Friedrich K, Pfausler B, Unterberger I, Matuja W, et al. A longitudinal study on nodding syndrome—A new African epilepsy disorder. Epilepsia. 2014;**55**(1):86-93

[55] Musisi S, Akena D. Neuropsychiatric perspectives on nodding syndrome in northern Uganda: A case series study and review of the literature. African Health Sciences. 2013;**13**(2):205-218

[56] MacFabe DF, Cain NE, Boon F, Ossenkopp KP, Cain DP. Effects of the enteric bacterial metabolic product propionic acid on object-directed behavior, social behavior, cognition, and neuro-inflammation in adolescent rats: Relevance to autism spectrum disorder. Behavioural Brain Research. 2011; **217**(1):47-54

[57] MacFabe DF, Cain DP, Rodriguez-Capote K, Franklin AE, Hoffman JE, Boon F, et al. Neurobiological effects of intraventricular propionic acid in rats: Possible role of short chain fatty acids on the pathogenesis and characteristics of autism spectrum disorders. Behavioural Brain Research. 2007; **176**(1):149-169

[58] Nicholson JK, Holmes E, Kinross J. Host-gut microbiota metabolic interactions. Science. 2012;**336**(6086): 1262-1267

[59] Patterson PH. Maternal infection and autism. Brain, Behavior, and Immunity. 2012;**26**(3):393

[60] Human Microbiome Project Consortium. Structure, function and diversity of the healthy human

microbiome. Nature. 2012;**486**(7402): 207-214

[61] Midtvedt AC, Midtvedt T. Production of short-chain fatty acids by the intestinal microflora during the first 2 years of human life. Journal of Pediatric Gastroenterology and Nutrition. 1992;**15**(4):395-403

[62] Yap IK, Angley M, Veselkov KA, Holmes E, Lindon JC, Nicholson JK. Urinary metabolic phenotyping differentiates children with autism from their unaffected siblings and age-matched controls. Journal of Proteome Research. 2010;**9**(6):2996-3004

[63] MacFabe DF, Rodriguez-Capote K, Hoffman JE. A novel rodent model of autism: Intraventricular infusions of propionic acid increase locomotor activity and induce neuro-inflammation and oxidative stress in discrete regions of adult rat brain. American Journal of Biochemistry and Biotechnology. 2008; **4**(2):146-166

[64] Thomas RH, Meeking MM, Mepham JR. The enteric bacterial metabolite propionic acid alters brain and plasma phospholipid molecular species: Further. Development of a rodent model of autism spectrum disorders. Journal of Neuroinflammation. 2012;**9**(1):153

[65] Barnevik-Olsson M, Gillberg C, Fernell E. Prevalence of autism in children of Somali origin living in Stockholm: Brief report of an at-risk population. Developmental Medicine and Child Neurology. 2010;**52**(12): 1167-1168

[66] Forsythe P, Sudo N, Dinan T, Taylor VH, Bienenstock J. Mood and gut feelings. Brain, Behavior, and Immunity. 2010;**24**(1):9-16

[67] Vargas DL, Nascimbene C, Krishnan C, Zimmerman AW, Pardo CA. Neuroglial activation and neuroinflammation in the brain of patients with autism. Annals of Neurology. 2005;**57**(1):67-81

[68] Chauhan A, Chauhan V. Oxidative stress in autism. Pathophysiology. 2006; **13**(3):171-181

[69] Kohman RA, Rhodes JS. Neurogenesis, inflammation and behavior. Brain, Behavior, and Immunity. 2013;**27**(1):22-32

[70] Brass EP, Beyerinck RA. Effects of propionate and carnitine on the hepatic oxidation of short- and medium-chain-length fatty acids. Journal of Biochemistry. 1988;**250**(3):819-825

[71] Frye RE. Biomarkers of abnormal energy metabolism in children with autism spectrum disorder. North American Journal of Medical Sciences. 2012;**5**(3):141-147

[72] Frye RE, Melnyk S, MacFabe DS. Unique acyl-carnitine profiles are potential biomarkers for acquired mitochondrial disease in autism spectrum disorder. Translational Psychiatry. 2013;**3**:e220. DOI: 10.1038/tp.2012.143

[73] Frye RE, Rossignol DA. Mitochondrial dysfunction can connect the diverse medical symptoms associated with autism spectrum disorders. Pediatric Research. 2011;**69**: 41R-47R

[74] Rossignol DA, Frye RE. Mitochondrial dysfunction in autism spectrum disorders: A systematic review and meta-analysis. Molecular Psychiatry. 2011;**25**(17):290-314

[75] El-Ansary AK, Ben BA, Kotb M. Etiology of autistic features: The persisting neurotoxic effects of propionic acid. Journal of Neuroinflammation. 2012;**9**(1):74

[76] Gottschall E. Breaking the Vicious Cycle: Intestinal Health through Diet.

Baltimore, Ontario, Canada: The Kirkton Press; 1994

[77] Wang L, Christophersen CT, Sorich MJ, Gerber JP, Angley MT, Conlon MA. Elevated fecal short chain fatty acid and ammonia concentrations in children with autism spectrum disorder. Digestive Diseases and Sciences. 2012; **57**(8):2096-2102

[78] Williams BL, Hornig M, Buie T. Impaired carbohydrate digestion and transport and mucosal dysbiosis in the intestines of children with autism and gastrointestinal disturbances. PLoS One. 2011;**6**(9):e24585

[79] Saulnier DM, Ringel Y, Heyman MB. The intestinal microbiome, probiotics and prebiotics in neurogastroenterology. Gut Microbes. 2013;**4**(1):17-27

[80] Cryan JF, Dinan TG. Mind-altering microorganisms: The impact of the gut microbiota on brain and behaviour. Nature Reviews. Neuroscience. 2012; **13**(10):701-712

[81] Suren P, Bakken IJ, Aase H, White RA, Bjornholt JV, Baird DD. Novel developmental analyses identify longitudinal patterns of early gut microbiota that affect infant growth. PLoS Computational Biology. 2013;**9**(5): e1003042

[82] Suren P, Bakken IJ, Aase H. Autism spectrum disorder, ADHD, epilepsy, and cerebral palsy in Norwegian children. Pediatrics. 2012;**130**(1):e152-e158

[83] Sokol MS. Infection-triggered anorexia nervosa in children: Clinical description of four cases. Journal of Child and Adolescent Psychopharmacology. 2000;**10**(2): 133-145

[84] Kerbeshian J, Burd L. Is anorexia nervosa a neuropsychiatric developmental disorder? An illustrative case report. The World Journal of Biological Psychiatry. 2009;**10**(4 Pt 2): 648-657

[85] Cho I, Yamanishi S, Cox L. Antibiotics in early life alter the murine colonic microbiome and adiposity. Nature. 2012;**488**(7413):621-626

[86] Petrof EO, Claud EC, Gloor GB, Allen-Vercoe E. Microbial ecosystems therapeutics: A new paradigm in medicine? Beneficial Microbes. 2013; **4**(1):53-65

[87] Diamond J. Guns, Germs, and Steel. New York, NY: W.W. Norton & Company, Inc; 1997

[88] Hoffman TL, Simon EM, Ficicioglu C. Biotinidase deficiency: The importance of adequate follow-up for an inconclusive newborn screening result. European Journal of Pediatrics. 2005; **164**:298-301

Chapter 3

Autism in the Classroom: Educational Issues across the Lifespan

Yasamin Bolourian, Katherine K.M. Stavropoulos and Jan Blacher

Abstract

This chapter reviews educational strategies and legal policies impacting effective schooling for children, youth, and young adults. Emphasis is on the classroom manifestation of autism spectrum disorder (ASD), and how general education teachers can effectively facilitate learning. Within early school years, the importance of positive student-teacher relationships (STRs) in the face of challenging behaviors is discussed, including ways to build positive STRs. In middle and high school, social relationships serve as protective factors against mental health problems (e.g., depression, anxiety). Literature on this topic, including issues related to bullying, is presented. In postsecondary settings, young adults with ASD continue to have poor outcomes (e.g. loneliness, unemployment); strategies for helping adolescents transition to adulthood is discussed. While there are many other aspects to educational program appropriate for individuals with ASD (e.g., curriculum content), this chapter highlights recent issues that may be informative to a wide audience—school teachers and staff, researchers, and parents.

Keywords: education, classroom, school-aged, transition, lifespan, autism

1. Introduction

While much has been learned about how to educate children with autism spectrum disorder (ASD), and program successes are widely touted, children and youth with ASD are nonetheless at heightened risk for poor academic outcomes, including conflictual relationships with general education teachers [1] and more restrictive classroom placement [2]. Such outcomes are likely due to the presence of substantial social difficulties that are inherent to the ASD diagnosis [3], as well as behavioral difficulties that children with ASD often display [2, 4]. Indeed, it has been documented that individuals with ASD have significantly higher behavior problems than those with intellectual disability and those with typical development [5]. These heightened externalizing and internalizing problems evident in ASD, as well as poorer social skills, may also place these young students at risk for poor long-term school adjustment [1, 6].

As almost half (44%) of students with ASD fall in the typical range or above on cognitive ability [7], it is not uncommon for these students to be placed into general education classrooms [8]. Indeed, placement in general education has been shown to be beneficial for many students with ASD [9] and is often preferred by parents, yet, general education teachers receive little specialized training on how to effectively manage students with ASD in the classroom. Moreover, many school districts are unprepared to accommodate such students, as evidenced by the number of legal disputes with families of students with ASD [10]. The purpose of this chapter is to discuss selected recent advances in research on autism in the classroom and educational issues in the context of ASD in the twenty-first century.

2. Educational issues

Issued in 2004, the *Individuals with Disabilities Education Improvement Act* (IDEA) mandated that educational programs for children with disabilities be delivered in the least restrictive environment (LRE). Inherent to the definition of LRE is the notion that a child with special needs should be educated in an environment containing same-aged typically developing peers. Many school districts have implemented a full-inclusion policy for young children with disabilities, including those receiving services for ASD [2], in order to comply with this mandate. These policies are not without challenges. Indeed, students with ASD have been documented to have the highest number of contested individualized education plans (IEPs) and educational rights litigation [10–14]. Nonetheless, some investigators have reported that the only disability group making progress towards spending more time in general education was students with ASD [15].

3. Placement

Students with ASD who are educated in a general education setting often experience greater success than students who are placed in special education classrooms [9]. Parents of children with ASD are generally in favor of inclusion. Leyser and Kirk [16] surveyed 437 parents of children with disabilities, including autism, and found that the following were related to a more positive parental disposition towards inclusion: (1) children with more mild disabilities, (2) parents with younger elementary school children, (3) parents with a college education, and (4) parents who did not know their child's educational placement. Moreover, White and colleagues [17] found that once the decision about placement had been determined, it rarely changed; students usually remained in that setting throughout their years of education. This further underscores the importance of helping schools and families make appropriate placement decisions in early school years; however, that decision can legally be revisited [18].

Research suggests that placement decisions for students with ASD may not necessarily be a function of student need. In order to examine the effects of school placement, Kurth and Mastergeorge [19] studied 15 students with ASD (12–15 years of age) who were enrolled in either an inclusive general education (n = 7) or special day class (n = 8). Although students enrolled in general education had a higher overall mean score in cognitive and adaptive functioning, this difference was not statistically significant, likely due to the small sample size.

Determinants of placement may also include beliefs and attitudes of school personnel [20, 21]. For example, in 2008, Horrocks and colleagues surveyed 571 principals in the Pennsylvania public schools. From a list of eleven principal characteristics (e.g., years in district, formal training, school level), there were two significant factors in predicting placement in regular education classrooms: the principals' experience working with students with autism and their beliefs that children with ASD could be included in general education. Praisner [21] also found that school principals often based their placement decisions on their experiences and beliefs. Specifically, students with ASD and those with emotional disturbance were least likely to be recommended for placement in an inclusion classroom.

Other studies indicate that placement may be determined by certain child characteristics. For example, Lauderdale-Littin, Howell, and Blacher [22] investigated differences between the characteristics of 56 children with ASD placed in public and non-public school settings. Logistic regression analyses indicated that child age, family income, and social skills were predictive of educational placement, such that older children from higher income households and who have lower levels of social skills were more likely to be placed in non-public, more restrictive school settings. The more obvious predictor of school placement is likely IQ or cognitive functioning; Harris and Handleman [23] reported that higher IQ and younger age at intake to an early intervention program were predictive of regular class placement upon the transition to school.

4. Role of the family at school

An understanding of family impact is a crucial foundation for general and special education teachers of children with ASD to build a strong partnership. Such alliances between parents and teachers are beneficial to children with ASD [24]. The quality of parent-teacher relationships appears to be an important force in the early school experiences of children with ASD [25, 26] and in later academic skill acquisition [27]. For example, in a study of 121 parents of young children with ASD [26], parents who had positive relationships with teachers had formed more positive expectations for the school year. However, it is important to note that when child behavior problems were entered into analyses, they uniquely predicted parent expectations. Moreover, parents with strong relationships with their child's teacher and who perceived the teacher to be warm and positive towards their child were less likely to end up in litigation [14, 28].

Disagreements regarding Individualized Education Plan (IEP) outcomes often contribute to the strain between parents and teachers. In a study of 142 parents of young children (ages 4–8 years) with ASD, a meaningful proportion of parents reported dissatisfaction with the IEP process [29]. Specifically, 41% of parents reported only some, or no, agreement between the IEP document and the services received. Parents' relationship with the teacher and school involvement, as reported by both parents and teachers, were positively associated with IEP satisfaction. Notably, family income and financial resources were also significantly related to IEP satisfaction, such that more resourced families tended to be more satisfied. Nevertheless, these findings highlight the importance of working with parents to increase consistency across the home and school context [30, 31].

5. Student-teacher relationships in early school years

The transition to early schooling is a crucial milestone for all children, one that can be particularly challenging for young children with ASD. The quality of the student-teacher relationship (STR) is seen as crucial to successful academic outcomes [32, 33] and a strong predictor of long-term behaviors [34–36]. For example, close, supportive relationships with teachers are associated with stronger social skills [37] and higher peer acceptance [38] in typically developing young children. However, on average, children with ASD experience poor relationships with their teachers as evidence by low closeness and high conflict [35, 39].

In order to examine the relations among social impairments, behavior problems, and STRs, Blacher and colleagues [1] conducted a comparison study of children (*M* age of 8 years) with ASD (*n* = 36), intellectual disability (ID; *n* = 38), and typical development (TD; *n* = 91). The measure used to assess STRs (*Student-Teacher Relationship Scale*; [40]) included domains of closeness, conflict, and dependency. Results revealed that students with ASD scored significantly lower on closeness and significantly higher on conflict than the ID or TD groups. Scores of dependency were statistically similar for both the ASD and ID groups but higher than that for the TD group. Moreover, closeness was accounted for mainly by social skills, while conflict was accounted for by behavior problems.

Currently, there are approximately 1,308,100 paraprofessionals or teacher aides employed; this number is expected to grow at the average rate of 8% by 2026 [41, 42]. The projected increase in paraprofessionals can be attributed to the demand of inclusive education, which may perpetuate an overreliance on their role in the school system [43]. Therefore, there is an immense need to support paraprofessionals in the instruction and behavior management of students with disabilities in inclusive environments [41]. Moreover, a heavy reliance on paraprofessionals creates fewer opportunities for teachers to develop close and supportive relationships with these students.

6. Middle and high school

Peer relationships seem to be the most salient issue for many middle and high school students with ASD. The lack of social skills that persists throughout adolescence has a negative impact on friendships and peer interactions [44]. In clinical populations, improvements in the social skills of children and adolescents with ASD are modest over time. Constantino and colleagues [45] examined the development of social skills at child ages 3 and 18 in a sample of 95 males without ASD and 85 males with pervasive developmental disorder. Results revealed that for the sample with clinical diagnoses, parent and teacher reports on the *Social Responsiveness Scale* (SRS; [46]) were correlated at both time points. While improvements were seen on the total SRS scores over time, these only reached significance in parent reports, leading the authors to conclude that social improvements over time were subtle or perhaps not obviously manifested in the school setting.

Enduring social difficulties have been found to lead to teasing and bullying by peers, more so for youth with ASD than their typically developing peers [47, 48]. Through interviews with early adolescents (age 13) with ASD, Zeedyk and colleagues [48] found that youth with ASD were victimized more frequently than youth with ID or TD. Above and beyond disability status, higher internalizing behavior problems and peer conflict were significant predictors of victimization. In 2018, Tipton-Fisler and colleagues did a follow-up study with the same youth at age 15 to explore how experiences of bullying and victimization changed for children with TD, ID, and ASD over time [47]. Consistent with Zeedyk et al., [48], they found that adolescents with ASD were bullied more frequently than those with ID or TD. Further, higher levels of internalizing behavior problems at age 13 related to higher levels of bullying at age 15.

These findings are consistent with previous research on internalizing behaviors in youth with ASD and victimization. Cappadocia and colleagues [49] found that internalizing behavior problems predicted victimization in a sample of youth with ASD. Whitehouse and colleagues [50] found that friendship conflicts were a significant predictor of depression in adolescents with ASD. Taken together, this body of research suggests a relationship between internalizing problems (e.g. depression, anxiety) and victimization and/or peer conflicts in youth with ASD. This work also underscores the importance of empirically supported interventions for youth with ASD who display internalizing behaviors. Such interventions could help youth make and keep friends, and provide information about how to deal with bullying. One example of such an intervention is the UCLA PEERS Program, which has a manualized curriculum designed to help youth with ASD make and keep friends, handle conflicts with friends, and bullying [51].

It is interesting that by middle or high school, students with ASD spend most of their time in a classroom with typically developing students, but interacting with other students with disabilities or with a paraprofessional, leaving few opportunities for socialization. Feldman and colleagues [52] demonstrated this in a study of high school youth. When they calculated the percent of time that students with ASD were present in the classroom, they found that, on average, that students with ASD were present for about 81% of a class period. When in class, students were in proximity to their peers in general education classrooms only for about a third (38%) of a class period.

7. Postsecondary school years

Unfortunately, difficulties for youth with ASD continue into young adulthood. According to a 2012 study, nearly 80% of young adults with ASD lived at home, 40% did not have contact with friends, and more than half (52%) did not have employment or postsecondary training 1–2 years after high school [53]. One possible reason for these dismal outcomes is the significant "service cliff" which occurs once young adults transition to independence. This is particularly notable after public school services end, for many as late as age 22 [18]. Thus, families of youth with ASD should prepare for the transition to postsecondary environments as early as possible. Geller and Greenberg [54] suggest that by age 14, planning should begin, and focus on areas of independence, including self-determination, functional skills, and social-communication skills needed for postsecondary life, especially for those young adults who have concomitant intellectual disability.

Approximately half of students with ASD are cognitively high functioning, with IQs in the typically developing range [7]; for them, attending college is a realistic goal. Predictors of college participation for young adults with ASD include student, family, and transition planning factors, such as attendance in a regular high school; strong academic performance in high school higher household income; parental expectations for attending college; post-secondary goals identified through transition planning; and student participation in transition planning [55].

Youth with ASD have at least two pathways to post-secondary education: [1] attending a 2-year school (community or junior college, depending on the state), or [2] attending a 4-year college or institution. In their review, Zeedyk, Tipton, and Blacher [56] highlighted some of the main benefits of 2- and 4-year institutions specifically for students with ASD. Two-year schools may provide more individualized supports, offer vocational programs, be more likely to be populated by familiar peers from high school, and provide weekly homework assignments similar to high school. On the other hand, 4-year schools usually offer more generic support services, a variety of programs, a more diverse curriculum, more majors to choose from, and sometimes a larger campus community.

Using the National Longitudinal Transition Study-2, a nationally representative dataset on young adults across 10 years, Sanford et al. [57] found that more young adults with ASD attended 2-year colleges than 4-year colleges (32 versus 17%). Moreover, the percentages of college attendance were statistically significantly lower for students with ASD than students with other types of disabilities. Lastly, only 39% of students with ASD graduated college, compared to 41% of students with disabilities in general and 52% of students from the typical population.

Given the dismal college attendance and completion rates, researchers have investigated some of the challenges students with ASD face in postsecondary environments that may impede their success in college. These factors include social difficulties which are related to the characteristics of ASD (e.g., [58]) and inhibit academic success. For example, students may have difficulty adapting to changing school schedules, to the complex social environment associated with college life, and to independent living responsibilities. Unfortunately, supports available in the college setting that focus on academic needs do not address the unique needs of young adults with ASD. Rather, they are generic and largely designed for students with learning disabilities. For example, typical academic accommodations in postsecondary settings may include extended test time, distraction free testing, flexible due dates for assignments, breaks during class, the use of technology in the classroom, note takers, and possibly optional group activities [56, 59].

However, the range of needs of young adults with ASD extend beyond academics critical to postsecondary success [60, 61]. Aside from social concerns, mental health issues are commonly found in ASD populations. Among college students, about 70–90% have reported symptoms of anxiety and/or depression. In a recent study by Jackson and colleagues [62], approximately 18% of students expressed wanting to attempt suicide in the future. Other associated difficulties in ASD include a lack of daily living skills, organization and planning, and flexibility [63]. These areas may be more stressful to cope with in the college environment, as students have less structure in their routines and less support from parents after high school. Some students with ASD also struggle with inappropriate classroom behavior in college (e.g., frequently raising one's hand, refusing to work in groups with classmates, calling out inappropriately).

Many of the challenges noted above are similar to other "invisible disorders," primarily attention-deficit/hyperactivity disorder (ADHD; [60, 64, 65]). For this reason, Bolourian and colleagues [60] conducted a qualitative study of 13 young adults with ASD and 18 students with ADHD in 4-year universities located in Southern California, to determine if young adults with ASD had challenges specific to their disorder. From coded in-depth interviews, nine themes emerged, highlighting the similar deficits between the two disorders. The authors also calculated passage frequencies to determine and compare how often these themes were discussed by members of each groups. While most themes did not statistically significantly differ, the theme of *Negative Peer Interactions* was unique to students with ASD, indicating that university staff need to do more to expand services for college students with ASD. In particular, supports and services to foster more positive social interactions on campus would be helpful, whether in the form of social skills groups conducted on campus, peer volunteers, or even group counseling sessions offered by disabilities services on campus.

7.1 Student-faculty relationships

Student-faculty relationships may also be impaired for college students with ASD. While student-teacher relationships are more frequently examined in early school years, poor relationship quality has been reported through secondary school for students without disabilities, particularly in relation to academic motivation [66, 67]. Thus, it is plausible that the quality of these relationships, even for youth with ASD, can endure into postsecondary environments.

Not surprisingly, many young adults on the spectrum enter postsecondary education with a passion for a particular subject area, which may inspire the selection of their major. Faculty awareness of these special areas of interest may help them to work this interest into course projects or requirements, thereby increasing student interest or focus. Of course, more interest can lead to better student performance, leading to higher grades, the likelihood of college graduation, and future employment. Thus, there is a rationale for faculty to be aware of their students with ASD and to foster the same type of academic relationship with them that they have with their other students.

There are many things faculty need to know in order to appropriately and comfortably teach and interact with students on the autism spectrum. In a survey of 132 faculty [68], a little over half of professors did not include a statement about disability services in their syllabus (55%), nor did they make a statement about services at the start of the quarter (60%). In terms of their beliefs about students with autism, 47% expected students to interact with peers in the classroom and 78% agreed that they would consider allowing students to work in their lab or on their research team. With regard to student disability services, 12% did not understand the role of disability service offices on campus, and 46% agreed that students with ASD should disclose their disability to disability services. These findings emphasize the importance of educating university faculty on ASD and providing resources on how to support students with ASD in their classrooms.

8. Resources available to educators

There are a number of resources available to teachers of children with ASD, particularly those at the early childhood or elementary levels. Many of these focus on intervention methods, and although classroom teachers may not be responsible for their implementation, understanding the evidence-base is useful as the greatest gains are made during the early school year [69]. Behavioral therapy continues to be supported in the literature as an effective intervention for individuals with ASD (e.g., [70, 71]).

8.1 Resources for K-12 and beyond

In 2014, the National Professional Development Center on Autism Spectrum Disorders (NPDC) and the Institute of Education Sciences funded a project to identify evidence-based practices (EBP) for individuals with ASD, from birth to 22 years [72]. This rigorous review yielded 27 practices, many of which are based on behavioral techniques, including reinforcement, naturalistic approaches, and self-management. While an update of this review is in progress, the NPDC created a free online curriculum that describes the key components of each identified EBP and provides a step-by-step approach to implementing these practices (i.e., Autism Focused Intervention Resources and Modules [AFIRM]; retrievable from https://afirm.fpg.unc.edu).

From the Ohio Center for Autism and Low-Incidence Disabilities, the Autism Internet Modules (AIM) is another free online training program (retrievable from www.autisminternetmodules.org). One way in which AIM differs from AFIRM is by its organization of material, centered around autism in the home, in the classroom, on the job, and in the community. The modules provide static content and interactive videos to highlight various evidence-based strategies that may be used across these settings.

8.2 Transitioning to the university

As research on the transition to postsecondary settings receives increasing attention, interventions aimed at supporting youth during these periods are being examined for their efficacy. For example, Lei and colleagues [73] implemented a 3-day, overnight summer school program in the UK for youth with ASD, ages 16 or older, who are preparing for university life. The curriculum included lessons on 'work' (i.e., experiencing a typical lecture, appropriate socialization between students and faculty/staff, and disclosure of diagnosis), 'rest' (i.e., stress reduction, management of anxiety, and the importance of physical wellbeing), and 'play' (i.e., on-campus clubs and societies, social outings, and informal social experiences). The program was facilitated by staff from the university's psychology department, disability office, and career services office; one session was facilitated by a current or recently graduated student with ASD. The program also offered the support of a 'student ambassador' or current typically-developing university student trained to provide broader support in inclusion activities. Findings from a satisfaction survey of 125 participating students revealed promising results. For example, pre- and post-program data showed significant changes on endorsed concerns associated with the transition to university, including in the areas of socialization, independence, and academic functioning. Moreover, on average, participants rated the program to be very enjoyable and helpful, and viewed going to university somewhat positively. With regard to the program components, students found psychoeducation (14.6%) and information on clubs and societies (11.5%) to be most helpful. With regard to their future at the university, students were most enthusiastic in their response about looking forward to new social opportunities (55.7%).

Mentoring has also been examined in the context of social-emotional supports for students with ASD in postsecondary environments. Lucas and James [74] tested the effect of a mentoring program for three undergraduate students with ASD and two with mental health conditions. After the first term, mentees with ASD expressed that mentors had been helpful for exam support, maintenance and development of social relationships, and promotion of positive well-being, while mentees with mental health issues did not find mentors as helpful in these areas. Other identified suggestions for social-emotional support include disability support groups, access to counseling, and private living spaces. However, isolation in private living spaces may also contribute to mental health issues. Thus, individualizing these supports is highly recommended and may consist of coupling accommodations (e.g., private living space and participation in mentorship program; [75]).

9. Conclusion: looking forward

Existing preparation programs for school administrators provide little knowledge considered necessary to understand the behaviors of students with ASD and implement inclusion programs [20, 76]. Teachers at the K-12 levels show wide variability in their ASD-specific knowledge and self-efficacy, with large numbers reporting a lack of training or readiness to teach students with ASD [72, 77]. However, the high incidence of ASD indicates that educators across the nation will inevitably encounter a student with ASD [78], underscoring the need to prepare special educators in evidence-based approaches that enhance the academic and social learning opportunities for these children [79]. With regard to the professional development of *university faculty* on ASD, research is still limited as to how to best help support faculty in accommodating students with ASD in their classrooms. It is clear that the development of a faculty training may be beneficial, as the volume of information available for how to best support these students may be overwhelming for professors to sift through themselves.

Acknowledgements

This paper was based on the activities of the Smooth Sailing Study, supported by the Institute of Education Sciences, Grant number R324A110086. We also appreciate the support from the SEARCH Family Autism Resource Center at UC Riverside and the UCR Vice Chancellor for Research.

Conflict of interest

Yasamin Bolourian, Katherine Stavropoulos, and Jan Blacher declare that they have no conflict of interest.

Author details

Yasamin Bolourian, Katherine K.M. Stavropoulos and Jan Blacher*
University of California, Riverside, CA, United States

*Address all correspondence to: jan.blacher@ucr.edu

References

[1] Blacher J, Howell E, Lauderdale-Littin S, Reed FDD, Laugeson EA. Autism spectrum disorder and the student teacher relationship: A comparison study with peers with intellectual disability and typical development. Research in Autism Spectrum Disorder. 2014;**8**(3):324-333

[2] Etscheidt S. Least restrictive and natural environments for young children with disabilities: A legal analysis of issues. Topics in Early Childhood Special Education. 2006;**26**(3):167-178

[3] Association AP. Diagnostic and Statistical Manual of Mental Disorders (DSM-5®). Washington, DC: American Psychiatric Pub; 2013

[4] Blacher J, Baker BL, Eisenhower AS. Student-teacher relationship stability across early school years for children with intellectual disability or typical development. American Journal on Intellectual and Developmental Disabilities. 2009;**114**(5):322-339

[5] Blacher J, Baker BL. Collateral effects of youth disruptive behavior disorders on Mothers' psychological distress: Adolescents with autism spectrum disorder, intellectual disability, or typical development. Journal of Autism and Developmental Disorders. 2017:1-12

[6] Eisenhower AS, Bush HH, Blacher J. Student-teacher relationships and early school adaptation of children with ASD: A conceptual framework. Journal of Applied School Psychology. 2015;**31**(3):256-296

[7] Christensen DL, Baio J, Van Naarden Braun K, Bilder D, Charles J, Constantino JN, et al. Prevalence and characteristics of autism spectrum disorder among children aged 8 years-autism and developmental disabilities monitoring network, 11 sites, United States, 2012. MMWR Surveillance Summaries. 2016;**65**(3):1-23

[8] Goodman G, Williams CM. Interventions for increasing the academic engagement of students with autism spectrum disorders in inclusive classrooms. Teaching Exceptional Children. 2007;**39**(6):53-61

[9] Kurth JA. Educational placement of students with autism: The impact of state of residence. Focus on Autism and Other Developmental Disabilities. 2014;**30**(4):249-256

[10] Bolourian Y, Tipton-Fisler LA, Yassine J. Special education placement trends: Least restrictive environment across five years in California. Contemporary School Psychology. 2018:1-10

[11] Iovannone R, Dunlap G, Huber H, Kincaid D. Effective educational practices for students with autism spectrum disorders. Focus on Autism and Other Developmental Disabilities. 2003;**18**(3):150-165

[12] Fogt JB, Miller DN, Zirkel PA. Defining autism: Professional best practices and published case law. Journal of School Psychology. 2003;**41**(3):201-216

[13] Zirkel PA. The autism case law: Administrative and judicial rulings. Focus on Autism and Other Developmental Disabilities. 2002;**17**(2):84-93

[14] Zirkel PA. Autism litigation under the IDEA: A new meaning of "disproportionality?". Journal of Special Education Leadership. 2011;**24**:92-103

[15] Morningstar ME, Kurth JA, Johnson PE. Examining national trends in

educational placements for students with significant disabilities. Remedial and Special Education. 2016;**38**(1):3-12

[16] Leyser Y, Kirk R. Evaluating inclusion: An examination of parent views and factors influencing their perspectives. International Journal of Disability, Development and Education. 2004;**51**(3):271-285

[17] White SW, Scahill L, Klin A, Koenig K, Volkmar FR. Educational placements and service use patterns of individuals with autism spectrum disorders. Journal of Autism and Developmental Disorders. 2007;**37**(8):1403-1412

[18] Individuals with Disabilities Education Improvement Act [IDEA]. Pub. L. No. PL108-446. 2004

[19] Kurth JA, Mastergeorge AM. Academic and Cognitive Profiles of Students with Autism: Implications for Classroom Practice and Placement. International Journal of Special Education [Internet]. 2010;**25**(2): 8-14. Available from: https://eric.ed.gov/?id=EJ890580

[20] Horrocks JL, White G, Roberts L. Principals' attitudes regarding inclusion of children with autism in Pennsylvania public schools. Journal of Autism and Developmental Disorders. 2008;**38**(8):1462-1473

[21] Praisner CL. Attitudes of elementary school principals toward the inclusion of students with disabilities. Exceptional Children. 2003;**69**(2):135-145

[22] Lauderdale-Littin S, Howell E, Blacher J. Educational placement for children with autism spectrum disorders in public and nonpublic school settings: The impact of social skills and behavior problems. Education and Training in Autism and Developmental Disabilities 2013;**48**:469-78

[23] Harris SL, Handleman JS. Age and IQ at intake as predictors of placement for young children with autism: A four- to six-year follow-up. Journal of Autism and Developmental Disorders. 2000;**30**(2):137-142

[24] Council NR. Educating Children with Autism. Washington, DC: National Academy Press, Committee on Educational Interventions for Children with Autism, Division of Behavioral and Social Sciences and Education; 2001

[25] Bennett-Conroy W. Engaging Parents of 8th Grade Students in Parent/Teacher Bidirectional Communication. 2011

[26] Bush HH, Cohen SR, Eisenhower AS, Blacher J. Parents' educational expectations for young children with autism spectrum disorder. Education and Training in Autism and Developmental Disabilities. 2017;**52**(4):357-368

[27] Powell DR, Son SH, File N, San Juan RR. Parent-school relationships and children's academic and social outcomes in public school pre-kindergarten. Journal of School Psychology. 2010;**48**(4):269-292

[28] Seligmann TJ. Rowley comes home to roast: Judicial review of autism special education disputes. UC Davis Journal of Juvenile Law and Policy. 2005;**9**:217

[29] Slade N, Eisenhower A, Carter AS, Blacher J. Satisfaction with individualized education programs among parents of young children with ASD. Exceptional Children. 2017;**84**(3):242-260

[30] Hume K, Loftin R, Lantz J. Increasing independence in autism spectrum disorders: A review of three focused interventions. Journal of Autism and Developmental Disorders. 2009;**39**(9):1329-1338

[31] Schutte J. Real life, real progress for children with autism spectrum disorders: Strategies for successful generalization in natural environments. Education and Treatment of Children. 2010;**33**(2):326-328

[32] Pianta R, Hamre B, Downer J, Burchinal M, Williford A, LoCasale-Crouch J, et al. Early childhood professional development: Coaching and coursework effects on indicators of children's school readiness. Early Education and Development. 2017;**28**(8):956-975

[33] Pianta RC, Stuhlman MW. Teacher-Child Relationships and Children's Success in the First Years of School. School Psychology Review. 2004;**33**(3):444-458

[34] Doumen S, Verschueren K, Buyse E, Germeijs V, Luyckx K, Soenens B. Reciprocal relations between teacher-child conflict and aggressive behavior in kindergarten: A three-wave longitudinal study. Journal of Clinical Child and Adolescent Psychology. 2008;**37**(3):588-599

[35] Eisenhower AS, Blacher J, Bush HH. Longitudinal associations between externalizing problems and student–teacher relationship quality for young children with ASD. Research in Autism Spectrum Disorder. 2015;**9**:163-173

[36] Hamre BK, Pianta RC. Early teacher-child relationships and the trajectory of children's school outcomes through eighth grade. Child Development. 2001;**72**(2):625-638

[37] Howes C, Phillipsen LC, Peisner-Feinberg E. The consistency of perceived teacher–child relationships between preschool and kindergarten. Journal of School Psychology. 2000;**38**(2):113-132

[38] Sette S, Spinrad T, Baumgartner E. Links among Italian preschoolers' socio-emotional competence, teacher-child relationship quality and peer acceptance. Early Education and Development. 2013;**24**(6):851-864

[39] Caplan B, Feldman M, Eisenhower A, Blacher J. Student-teacher relationships for young children with autism spectrum disorder: Risk and protective factors. Journal of Autism and Developmental Disorders. 2016;**46**(12):3653-3666

[40] Pianta RC. Student-Teacher Relationship Scale: Professional Manual. Odessa, FL: Psychological Assessment Resources, Inc; 2001

[41] Irvin DW, Ingram P, Huffman J, Mason R, Wills H. Exploring paraprofessional and classroom factors affecting teacher supervision. Research in Developmental Disabilities. 2018;**73**:106-114

[42] Bureau of Labor Statistics USDoL. Occupational Outlook Handbook, Teacher Assistants. Available from: https://www.bls.gov/ooh/education-training-and-library/teacher-assistants.htm

[43] Giangreco MF, Smith CS, Pinckney E. Addressing the paraprofessional dilemma in an inclusive school: A program description. Research and Practice for Persons with Severe Disabilities. 2006;**31**(3):215-229

[44] Magiati I, Tay XW, Howlin P. Cognitive, language, social and behavioural outcomes in adults with autism spectrum disorders: A systematic review of longitudinal follow-up studies in adulthood. Clinical Psychology Review. 2014;**34**(1):73-86

[45] Constantino JN, Abbacchi AM, Lavesser PD, Reed H, Givens L, Chiang L, et al. Developmental course of autistic social impairment in males. Development and Psychopathology. 2009;**21**(1):127-138

[46] Constantino JN, Gruber CP. The Social Responsiveness Scale Manual. California: Western Psychological Services; 2005

[47] Tipton-Fisler LA, Rodriguez G, Zeedyk SM, Blacher J. Stability of bullying and internalizing problems among adolescents with ASD, ID, or typical development. Research in Developmental Disabilities. 2018;**80**:131-141

[48] Zeedyk S, Rodriguez G, Tipton L, Baker B, Blacher J. Bullying of youth with autism spectrum disorder, intellectual disability, or typical development: Victim and parent perspectives. Research in Autism Spectrum Disorder. 2014;**8**(9):1173-1183

[49] Cappadocia MC, Weiss JA, Pepler D. Bullying experiences among children and youth with autism spectrum disorders. Journal of Autism and Developmental Disorders. 2012;**42**(2):266-277

[50] Whitehouse AJO, Durkin K, Jaquet E, Ziatas K. Friendship, loneliness and depression in adolescents with asperger's syndrome. Journal of Adolescence. 2009;**32**(2):309-322

[51] Laugeson EA, Frankel F, Gantman A, Dillon AR, Mogil C. Evidence-based social skills training for adolescents with autism spectrum disorders: The UCLA PEERS program. Journal of Autism and Developmental Disorders. 2012;**42**(6):1025-1036

[52] Feldman R, Carter EW, Asmus J, Brock ME. Presence, proximity, and peer interactions of adolescents with severe disabilities in general education classrooms. Exceptional Children. 2015;**82**(2):192-208

[53] Shattuck PT, Narendorf SC, Cooper B, Sterzing PR, Wagner M, Taylor JL. Postsecondary education and employment among youth with an autism spectrum disorder. Pediatrics. 2012;**129**(6):1042-1049

[54] Geller LL, Greenberg M. Managing the transition process from high school to college and beyond: Challenges for individuals, families, and society. Social Work in Mental Health. 2009;**8**(1):92-116

[55] Chiang HM, Cheung YK, Hickson L, Xiang R, Tsai LY. Predictive factors of participation in postsecondary education for high school leavers with autism. Journal of Autism and Developmental Disorders. 2012;**42**(5):685-696

[56] Zeedyk SM, Tipton LA, Blacher J. Educational supports for high functioning youth with ASD: The postsecondary pathway to college. Focus on Autism and Other Developmental Disabilities. 2014;**31**(1):37-48

[57] Sanford C, Newman L, Wagner M, Knokey A-M, Marder C, Nagle K, et al. The post-high school outcomes of young adults with disabilities up to 8 years after high school. In: A Report from the National Longitudinal Transition Study-2 (NLTS2) (NCSER 2011-3005). Menlo Park, CA; 2011

[58] Volkmar FR, Jackson SLJ, Hart L. Transition issues and challenges for youth with autism spectrum disorders. Pediatric Annals. 2017;**46**(6):e219-ee23

[59] Van Hees V, Moyson T, Roeyers H. Higher education experiences of students with autism Spectrum disorder: Challenges, benefits and support needs. Journal of Autism and Developmental Disorders. 2015;**45**(6):1673-1688

[60] Bolourian Y, Zeedyk SM, Blacher J. Autism and the university experience: Narratives from students with neurodevelopmental disorders. Journal of Autism and Developmental Disorders. 2018

[61] Gelbar NW, Shefyck A, Reichow B. A comprehensive survey of current and former college students with autism spectrum disorders. Yale Journal of Biology and Medicine. 2015;**88**(1):45-68

[62] Jackson SLJ, Hart L, Brown JT, Volkmar FR. Brief report: Self-reported academic, social, and mental health experiences of post-secondary students with autism Spectrum disorder. Journal of Autism and Developmental Disorders. 2018;**48**(3):643-650

[63] Demetriou EA, Lampit A, Quintana DS, Naismith SL, Song YJC, Pye JE, et al. Autism spectrum disorders: A meta-analysis of executive function. Molecular Psychiatry. 2018;**23**(5):1198-1204

[64] Elias R, White SW. Autism Goes to college: Understanding the needs of a student population on the rise. Journal of Autism and Developmental Disorders. 2018;**48**(3):732-746

[65] Mayes SD, Calhoun SL, Mayes RD, Molitoris S. Autism and ADHD: Overlapping and discriminating symptoms. Research in Autism Spectrum Disorder. 2012;**6**(1):277-285

[66] Ryan RM, Stiller JD, Lynch JH. Representations of relationships to teachers, parents, and friends as predictors of academic motivation and self-esteem. Journal of Early Adolescence. 1994;**14**(2):226-249

[67] Fraire M, Longobardi C, Prino LE, Sclavo E, Settanni M. Examining The Student-Teacher Relationship Scale in the Italian Context: A Factorial Validity Study. Electronic Journal of Research in Educational Psychology. Dec 2013;**11**(3):851-882

[68] Zeedyk SM, Bolourian Y, Blacher J. University life with ASD: Faculty knowledge and student needs. Autism. 2018. DOI: 10.1177/1362361318774148

[69] Marsh A, Spagnol V, Grove R, Eapen V. Transition to school for children with autism spectrum disorder: A systematic review. World Journal of Psychiatry. 2017;**7**(3):184-196

[70] Vismara LA, Rogers SJ. Behavioral treatments in autism spectrum disorder: What do we know? Annual Review of Clinical Psychology. 2010;**6**:447-468

[71] Warren Z, McPheeters ML, Sathe N, Foss-Feig JH, Glasser A, Veenstra-Vanderweele J. A systematic review of early intensive intervention for autism spectrum disorders. Pediatrics. 2011;**127**(5):e1303-e1311

[72] Wong C, Odom SL, Hume KA, Cox AW, Fettig A, Kucharczyk S, et al. Evidence-based practices for children, youth, and young adults with autism spectrum disorder: A comprehensive review. Journal of Autism and Developmental Disorders. 2015;**45**(7):1951-1966

[73] Lei J, Calley S, Brosnan M, Ashwin C, Russell A. Evaluation of a transition to university programme for students with autism spectrum disorder. Journal of Autism and Developmental Disorders. 2018:1-15

[74] Lucas R, James AI. An evaluation of specialist mentoring for university students with autism Spectrum disorders and mental health conditions. Journal of Autism and Developmental Disorders. 2018;**48**(3):694-707

[75] MacLeod A, Green S. Beyond the books: Case study of a collaborative and holistic support model for university students with Asperger syndrome. Studies in Higher Education. 2009;**34**(6):631-646

[76] Wood P, Evans D, Spandagou I. Attitudes of principals towards students with disruptive behaviour: An

Australian perspective. Australasian Journal of Special Education. 2014;**38**(1):14-33

[77] Loiacono V, Valenti V. General education teachers need to be prepared to co-teach the increasing number of children with autism in inclusive settings. International Journal of Special Education. 2010;**25**(3):24-32

[78] Blacher J, Linn RH, Zeedyk SM. The role of graduate schools of education in training autism professionals to work with diverse families. In: Professional Responsibility. Switzerland: Springer; 2015. pp. 231-246

[79] Conroy MA, Alter PJ, Boyd BA, Bettini E. Teacher preparation for students who demonstrate challenging behaviors. In: Handbook of Research on Special Education Teacher Preparation. New York: Routledge; 2014. pp. 320-333

Chapter 4

The Effect of Scalp Acupuncture on Autism: Could This Be a Possible Treatment of Autism?

Chuen Heung Yau, Cheuk Long Ip, Yuk Yin Chau and Ho Cheung Lai

Abstract

No current conventional treatment methods have been proven effective in improving core symptoms of autism spectrum disorders (ASD). In pursuit of a potent remedy for ASD, scalp acupuncture, one of the complementary and alternative medicines (CAM), may have potential in treating children with ASD according to recent clinical studies. In our first study, the effect of scalp acupuncture on prominent symptoms of ASD was investigated. Factors contributing to the effectiveness of ASD such as age and onset pattern had also been evaluated. Results showed that verbal communication and social and behavioral aspects of the patient could benefit from scalp acupuncture. Moreover, early intervention before 3 years old will bring about better therapeutic outcomes. The effect of scalp acupuncture on emotional and behavioral problems in children with ASD was further elaborated in the second study. Our observation on patients noted drastic improvements in emotional and emotion-related behavioral problems after the introduction of scalp acupuncture. Feedbacks from parents also reflected a positive progress in performance on cognitive, social, and behavioral aspects after treatment. The influence of scalp acupuncture on the sleeping quality and habit in children with ASD was investigated in the third study. Children had shown less resistance and anxiety toward sleep after scalp acupuncture.

Keywords: effect, scalp acupuncture, treatment, autism, clinical study

1. Introduction

The prevalence of autism spectrum disorders (ASD) has been rising over the past 50 years. In 2017, statistics from WHO showed that one in every 160 children suffer from ASD [1]. The diagnosis of ASD emphasizes on specific presentations and malfunctions in various areas, including reciprocal social interaction, communication, and restricted and repetitive behaviors [2, 3].

Despite ASD being generally recognized as an incurable disease, numerous treatments have claimed to bring about major improvements or even recovery in autism. Various complementary and alternative medicine (CAM) treatments have been practiced to treat ASD. A study carried out in the United States reported that 74% of the children diagnosed with autism have ever tried one or more than one type of CAM treatments [4]. Among all the CAM available, scalp acupuncture has been widely used for treating ASD in Hong Kong and China. In a treatment of scalp acupuncture, needles are inserted onto specific acupoints in accordance with different lines or zones of the scalp.

At present, a number of randomized controlled trials had been carried out to investigate the use of acupuncture in treating autism [5]. Despite present statistical evidence remaining inconclusive, there is no lack of subjective clinical reports and preliminary data to support the uses of acupuncture in improving communication, linguistic ability, cognitive and global functioning of ASD patients [5, 6].

The presentation of ASD could be observed in the early months of the children as they may manifest abnormal social development and speech delay before 1 year old. They are recognized as early-onset or natal autism [7]. On the other hand, a portion of children might obtain normal development in their first 18 months before losing previously acquired skills. This type of onset pattern is named as regressive or acquired autism [8]. We tried to relate the familial and personal allergic history and the onset pattern of the children.

A successive study has been made in the area of the effect of scalp acupuncture on emotion and behavioral functioning in those children. Despite behavioral problems having been evaluated in the first study, we had not distinguished emotion related behavior from restricted repetitive behavior. Studies have suggested that patients with ASD display more emotion deregulation than normal children [9]. Emotion disturbance always results in behavioral problems such as aggression, tantrums, and self-injurious behavior or comorbidity with other mental disorders like anxiety [10]. Currently few studies have been made in evaluating the use of scalp acupuncture in alleviating emotion and behavioral problems. Indeed we were impressed with how effective scalp acupuncture is in moderating emotion and its manifestation of children with ASD in our clinical observation.

Another area that has aroused our interest is the sleeping quality and habit in children with ASD. Previous studies have shown that children with ASD are more likely to have comorbidity with sleeping disorders. And the relationship between sleep and cognitive function has been evaluated [11]. Studies have shown that better sleeping quality may advocate better improvement in the symptomatology [12]. Since acupuncture has been vastly used in treating sleep disorder in adolescents and adults in certain cultures, we hypothesize that ASD children with similar sleep problems may as well benefit from scalp acupuncture.

2. Subjects and methods

2.1 Participants

Children with ASD consulted for acupuncture treatment at Hong Kong Baptist University Mr. & Mrs. Chan Hon Yin Chinese Medicine Specialty Clinic and Good Clinical Practice Centre were invited to join the studies. Eligibility criteria included children of both gender, aged 2–11 years old. All participants were required to present a current medical document on the diagnosis of ASD issued by recognized specialist such as pediatrician, psychiatrist, or psychologist.

In the first study, 68 patients with autism spectrum disorders participated; there were 11 female and 57 male. Ages ranged from 2.1 to 10.6 years old (mean = 4.2 years old) 47 (69%) natal autism cases and 21 (31%) regressive autism cases were included.

In the second study, 45 participants joined the program, consisting of 35 males and 10 females. Ages ranged from 2 to 10 years old (mean = 3.8 years old).

In the third study, 21 participants were invited to the investigation, including 20 males and 1 female. Age ranges from 2 to 10.1 years old (mean = 3.91 years old).

2.2 Therapist and treatment

All clinical assessment and scalp acupuncture treatment sessions were performed by principal investigator (Yau Chuen Heung), who is a registered Chinese medicine practitioner and has been performing scalp acupuncture for children with ASD and other developmental disorders for 18 years in Hong Kong.

The therapist and the treatment procedure were identical in the three studies. In each treatment session, the participants in the treatment group first sat on a chair or positioned in the bosom of their parents. Their scalps were then sterilized with a 75% alcohol cotton ball before acupuncture needles were obliquely inserted onto the selected acupoints with the depth of 10 mm into the subcutaneous tissue. The choice of acupoints included the BaiHui (GV20), SiShenChong (EX-NH3), midline of forehead, lateral line two of forehead, posterior lateral line of vertex, primary auditory cortex, and auditory speech area. The standard of needles used was 0.20 × 25 mm. Needles were swirled at intervals of 15 minutes before they were carefully removed and discarded after 60 minutes. Treatment sessions were performed twice a week and involved 30 sessions in the whole course.

2.3 Measurement of outcome

At the time participants joined the study, their past medical history and demographic information was recorded in an assessment session. Materials concerning the onset of ASD and familial and personal history of allergic diseases were also collected and manipulated in the first study. Participants who lose the previously acquired language skills were categorized into regression group, otherwise will be included into the natal group.

In the first study, in order to evaluate the overall performance of the participants, they were assessed by a parent-rated inventory adjusted childhood autism rating scale (CARS). We designed a set of rating scale for quantifying symptoms of ASD. The evaluated items covered social problem, verbal communication problem, behavioral problems, food selectivity, and noise sensitivity. The inventory was completed at the time (a) before scalp acupuncture treatment and (b) after 30 sessions of treatment.

In the second study, we utilized a parent questionnaire which was established in reference to autism behavior checklist (ABC) that covers five items of behavioral problems commonly found in child with ASD, which are temper tantrum, aggression to others, self-injury, impatience, and fears and anxiety. The checklist was finished at time (a) before scalp acupuncture treatment and (b) after 30 sessions of treatment. The marking scheme for refined CARS and ABC is listed on **Table 1**.

In the third study, a children sleeping habit questionnaire (CSHQ) was filled by parents to evaluate the sleep-related performance at the time (a) 6 months before receiving scalp acupuncture, (b) at the beginning of the treatment, and (c) after 6 months of treatment. CSHQ consists of 33 questions categorized into 8 domains, including bedtime resistance, sleep anxiety, sleep-onset delay, sleep waking, sleep-disordered breathing, parasomnia, daytime sleepiness, and night waking. Parents are required to record the frequency of the respective items which occurred in their children in the previous 2 weeks. A score will be marked according the frequency of the items.

Score	Marking Criteria
0	No symptoms
1	Minimal symptoms, seldom shown
2	Mild symptoms, often shown
3	Moderate symptoms, usually shown
4	Severe symptoms, always shown

Table 1.
Marking criteria for childhood autism rating scale (CARS) and autism behavior checklist (ABC).

Data analyses were conducted on all treatment responders. An alpha level of 0.05 was used for all statistical tests. The alteration in the score of CARS, ABC, and CSHQ throughout the studies was analyzed using paired t-test and analyses of variance (ANOVAs). The influence of age to the therapeutic effect was evaluated by means of independent t-test and ANOVAs. Pearson chi-square tests were utilized to show the correlation among onset patterns of ASD, personal history of allergic disorder, and family history of allergy. Calculations and analyses were performed on software IBM SPSS Statistics (Windows, version 21).

3. Results

In the first study, we investigated the effect of acupuncture on the general presentation of ASD patients (**Table 2** and **Figure 1**). Background performance before treatment scored highest in verbal communication problems, followed by social problems and behavioral problems. In comparison, the presentation of food selectivity and noise sensitivity problems seem to be less prominent issues.

A significant improvement across all items was observed after 30 sessions of scalp acupuncture treatment ($p < 0.05$). Among all domains, improvement made on social problems and verbal communication problems has been most prominent. Other items such as behavioral problems, food selectivity, and noise sensitivity showed relatively less effective toward acupuncture treatment.

In the later section of the first study, we tried to observe how the age of the children influence the effect of the treatment. The result was shown on **Figure 2**.

	Pre-treatment		Post-treatment		
Items	Mean	SD	Mean	SD	P-value
All	11.46	2.37	8.29	2.03	.000
Verbal communication Problems	3.06	1.01	2.00	0.90	.000
Social problems	2.50	0.78	1.60	0.69	.000
Behavorial problems	2.34	1.07	1.72	0.77	.000
Food selectivity	1.85	0.70	1.49	0.63	.000
Noise sensitivity	1.71	0.88	1.49	0.76	.003

Table 2.
Performance in selected items in childhood autism rating scale (CARS) before and after the scalp acupuncture treatment.

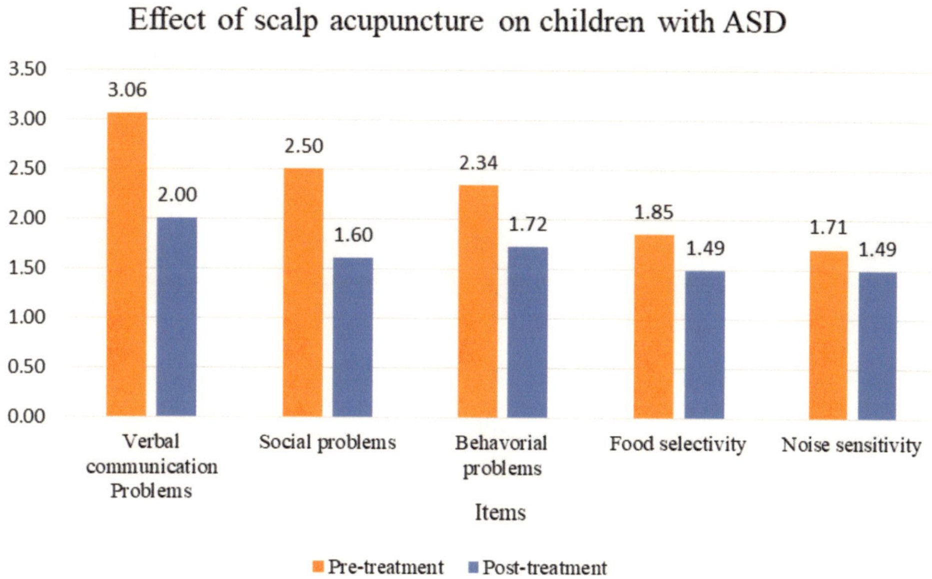

Figure 1.
Performance in selected items in childhood autism rating scale (CARS) before and after the scalp acupuncture treatment.

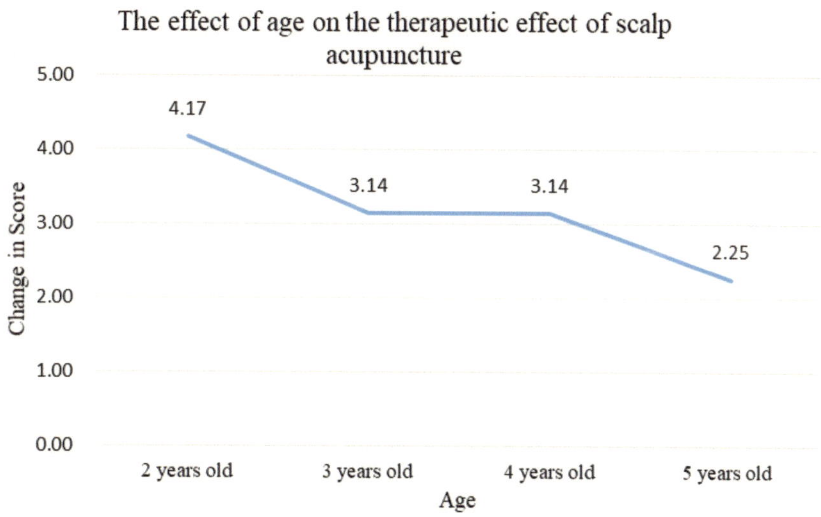

Figure 2.
The effect of age of the children on the therapeutic effect of scalp acupuncture treatment.

There is a significant downward trend of improvement along with an increase of age of the patients. Young children are more responsive to the scalp acupuncture and benefit more from the treatment, which cohere with our clinical observation.

The collected data obtained was further analyzed as we were interested in how regressive and natal-onset pattern varies in clinical presentation. Although no correlation between onset pattern and symptom severity could be established ($p > 0.05$), the familial occurrence of allergy disorder was found to closely related to the onset of ASD. Seventeen (25%) participants had shown various degree of allergic disorders such as allergic rhinitis, asthma, and eczema, while the remaining (75%) showed no history or relevant disorders. Around 29.4% ($n = 20$) participants' father or mother had a history of respiratory or dermatologic allergic disorder, while the rest of 70.6% (n = 48) participants' parents did not. Further analyses revealed a significant correlation between family and personal history of allergy diseases ($p = 0.000$) and between family history of allergies and the onset type of ASD ($p = 0.000$). On the contrary, the factor of personal history of allergies had shown irrelevance to the onset pattern of ASD ($p = 0.293$).

In the second study, we focused on how scalp acupuncture can help with emotion and emotion-related behavioral problem in children with ASD. Comparing the score of ABC inventory before and after treatment, items in temper tantrum, aggression to others, impatience, and fears and anxiety received a significant positive progress with a range of 0.53–0.29 points ($p < 0.05$), whereas the alteration in the scoring of self-injury was blunt ($p > 0.05$). Individuals generally showed less frequent occurrence and milder presentation of temper tantrum, aggression, impatience, and anxiety after scalp acupuncture. However, the presentation of self-injurious actions did not show significant response toward treatment (**Table 3** and **Figure 3**).

	Pre-treatment		Post-treatment		
Items	Mean	SD	Mean	SD	P-value
Temper tantrum	1.53	1.06	1.00	0.80	.000
Aggression to others	0.96	1.19	0.53	0.89	.015
Self injury	0.33	0.64	0.24	0.48	.209
Impatience	1.96	1.00	1.53	0.97	.009
Fears and anxiety	0.78	0.97	0.49	0.69	.022

Table 3.
Performance in selected items in autism behavior checklist (ABC) before and after the scalp acupuncture treatment.

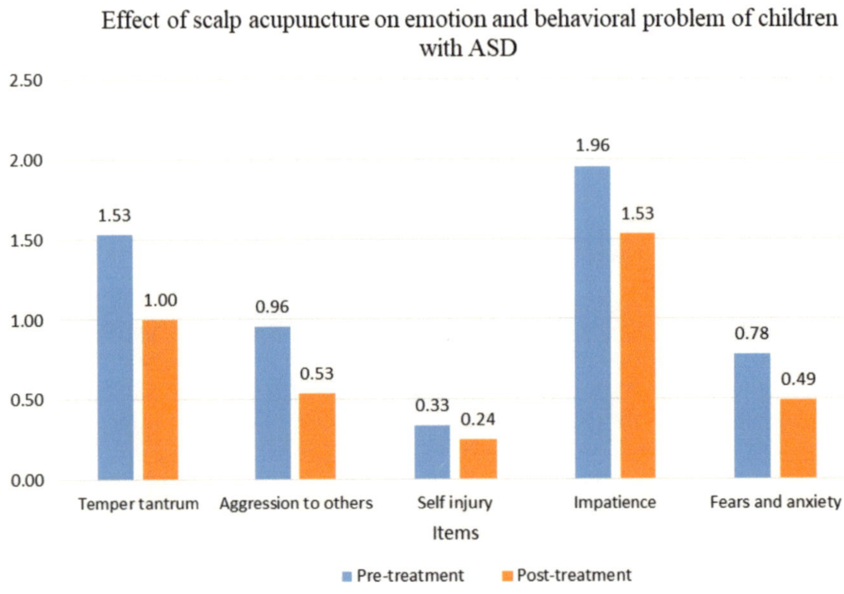

Figure 3.
Performance in selected items in autism behavior checklist (ABC) before and after the scalp acupuncture treatment.

Items	6 months prior to treatment			After 6 months of treatment		
	Mean	SD	P-value	Mean	SD	P-value
Total score	1.62	3.80	0.07	3.71	6.46	0.02
Bedtime resistance	0.48	1.83	0.25	0.90	1.34	0.01
Sleep onset delay	0.10	0.54	0.43	0.14	0.65	0.33
Sleep duration	0.19	0.75	0.26	0.33	1.11	0.18
Sleep anxiety	0.24	0.77	0.17	0.67	1.24	0.02
Sleep wakings	0.38	1.07	0.12	-0.14	1.28	0.61
Parasomnia	0.24	1.26	0.40	0.43	1.33	0.15
Sleep disordered breathing	0.24	0.62	0.10	0.29	0.96	0.19
Daytime sleepiness	-0.52	1.29	0.08	1.29	2.63	0.04

Table 4.
Comparison of the change in score of children sleeping habit questionnaire (CSHQ) between 6 months before treatment and after 6 months of scalp acupuncture treatment.

Our third study concerns about how scalp acupuncture alleviates sleeping problems encountered by children with ASD. The alteration in score of the eight subscales in the time periods "6 months prior to treatment" and "after 6 months of treatment" was shown in **Table 4**. The presentation in domains of bedtime resistance, sleep anxiety, and daytime sleepiness has shown significant improvement ($p < 0.05$) after 6 months of scalp acupuncture. In addition, we also observed an obvious decrease in the occurrence of nightmares reported after the introduction of the treatment ($p < 0.05$). However, no significant alteration was observed in the subscale of sleep-onset delay, night duration, sleep-disordered breathing, parasomnia, and sleep wakings.

4. Discussion

There are few theories proposed to explain the mechanism of scalp acupuncture on children with autism. Investigations had shown that acupuncture at the scalp can induce changes in perfusion in different brain areas. Biochemical alterations have also been noticed in individuals with ASD as they showed imbalances in level of catecholamine in blood and inside brain structures [13]. Acupuncture could correct and modulate respective catecholamine level [14]. Scalp acupuncture was observed to be able to improve defective brainwaves in brain diseases, which may also be applicable to children with ASD [15].

Theoretically, different areas and lines can be drawn on the scalp as a projection of functional areas of the cerebrum according to reflexology. Thus acupuncture at these areas was performed in order to stimulate the activity of the corresponding cerebral function. For example, the midline and the lateral line 2 of the forehead are in response to the prefrontal cortex of frontal lobes, posterior lateral line of vertex in response to posterior parietal lobe, auditory speech area in response to the Brodmann area 22, etc. We perceived that improvements in the cognitive ability such as verbal communication and social problems are more outstanding than sensory functions like sound sensitivity. Since hypoperfusion and the consequential underdevelopment at the inferior portion of prefrontal lobe and left temporal speech area could be detected in individuals with ASD, malnourishment at these areas contribute to defects in language abilities, communication problems, and retarded cognitive development [16]. Scalp acupuncture can induce better perfusion to these structures, thus bringing prospective progress in cognitive and communication development. On the contrary, the etiology of sensory dysfunction in ASD varies, result in differential responses among different developmental domains.

Moreover, auditory functioning in newborns becomes well-performed within days after labor. Infants are capable of discriminating sound frequency and intensity and making directional responses to sound at the first 3–6 months of age [17]. The rapid progress in gustatory and olfactory system provides infants with delicate sensory toward foods as early as they are 4–5 months old [18]. The early establishment of these sensory domains implies limited plasticity in altering the existing defective system by the time ASD is treated. In contrast, children develop language abilities at a slower rate for years before completing an effective communication system. The long duration of language and cognitive development with active neuroplasticity allows wider time window for receiving effective treatments.

Brain development continues to progress after birth through adolescence into Adulthood. It is most rapid in the first few years postnatal, given the fact that rate of increment in volume of white matter and gray matter in the cerebral cortex is the steepest during the first 2 and 4 years, respectively [19]. It may explain why children with age < 3 receive greater general therapeutic outcome from scalp acupuncture.

Strong correlation between familial or maternal atopic history and ASD has been well-recognized [20–23]. Molloy revealed familial autoimmune disease such as thyroid disease is a significant risk factor to the regressive onset of ASD [24]. Our investigation hints that familial atopies apart from thyroid disease, such as asthma, rhinitis, and eczema, also exhibit similar relationships.

Aggression and temper tantrum are commonly present in typically developing children. Children with psychiatric disorders, including ASD, have shown to have more aggressive behaviors and express exacerbated temper tantrums with greater emotional arousal lasting for longer period of time [25, 26]. After scalp acupuncture treatment, children with ASD might become gentler in temperament, their anger would be presented in a lower degree, and the duration of distress became shorter. Some children may even develop alternative coping strategies such as self-distraction and autosuggestion during stressful or undesirable events. We suggested that routine treatment sessions might pose a function of regular "emotion training," allowing the children to develop volitional regulation of affects. Apart from the psychological point of view, physiological investigations have suggested structural and biochemical aspects of the brain which also contributes to the mental activity. Exaggerated temper tantrum, aggressive, or even violent behaviors have been related to the frontal (mainly ventromedial frontal and orbitofrontal cortex) and temporal lobe abnormalities, implying damages in the area or reduction in tissue volume and activities. A distinct dysfunction at the anterior cingulate cortex (ACC) was perceived in children with conduct misbehaviors using functional magnetic resonance imaging (fMRI) [27]. It was also recognized as the place where acupuncture exerts its effect [28]. Biochemical basis of ASD has also been intensively studied. Patients with ASD often feature with hyperserotonemia conditions, resulting in unstable temperament and aggressive behaviors of an individual [29]. Since acupuncture was suggested to deliver its therapeutic effect by regulating serotonin level, it may explain how acupuncture brings about alteration in mood and behaviors of ASD individuals [14].

Concerning about the effect of scalp acupuncture on the performance of sleep in children with ASD, prominent improvements have been shown on items which are associated with emotional and behavioral components, i.e., bedtime resistance and anxiety. We suggest the effect of the treatment to be the consequence of the ameliorated emotion and behavior problems. Surprisingly, distressing and prominent sleep problems commonly found in children with ASD including irregular sleep-wake patterns or sleep wakings did not response well toward scalp acupuncture therapy. Neurobiological studies have suggested the aberration in neurotransmitter systems, including gamma-aminobutyric acid (GABA), serotonin, and melatonin, may be responsible for sleep disturbance in ASD [30]. Regarding the complexity and interactive nature of the contributing biological, psychological, and environmental factors in ASD [31], although acupuncture was proposed to be capable of modulating the deviated neurotransmitter system [32], no obvious improvement on circadian abnormalities has been detected in this study.

Although our studies showed encouraging outcomes in using scalp acupuncture on children with ASD, enormous efforts are required to further evaluate its clinical application and to understand the underlying mechanism. Since no comparison or controlled group was used in these studies, further randomized controlled trials are desirable. High-quality trials of larger sample size and longer follow-up period are needed to provide objective and definitive evidences on the therapeutic value of scalp acupuncture treatment on patients with ASD.

5. Conclusion

According to our preliminary studies, ASD manifestations of some aspects such as verbal communication, social, and behavioral problems may obtain significant improvement upon the introduction of acupuncture, whereas domains of food selectivity and auditory sensitivity benefit less in the process. Scalp acupuncture may also be effective in alleviating temper tantrum and aggression problems in children with ASD. It can facilitate emotion regulation on anger and diminish the frequency and the intensity of the related behavior. Comorbid sleep disorders likewise benefit from scalp acupuncture. The domains of bedtime resistance, sleep anxiety, daytime sleepiness, and nightmare have shown significant amelioration upon the introduction of the treatment.

Age is a predictor for the therapeutic effect of acupuncture. Early intervention is always encouraged for ASD children. Moreover, a significantly greater proportion of regressive-onset ASD patients shared positive familial allergy history than natal-onset ASD. Correlation between family history of atopy and onset type stated the difference in the nature of natal and regressive ASD.

Despite the rapid development of modern science, the incidence rate of ASD shows no sign of decline and ASD remains to be an incurable disorder. Only if we could reveal factors that contribute to the onset of ASD, preventive measures or effective treatments could be applied. Besides, further investigations are required in order to reveal the underlying mechanism of acupuncture, i.e., the psychological and physiologic effect of scalp acupuncture on children with ASD.

Acknowledgements

We would like to express our sincere gratitude to all people who have been associated with the projects. We thank all autistic patients and their parents for their cooperation. Also thanks go to School of Chinese Medicine, Hong Kong Baptist University for supporting the projects.

List of abbreviations

ABC	autism behavior checklist
ACC	anterior cingulate cortex
ASD	autism spectrum disorders

CAM	complementary and alternative medicine
CARS	childhood autism rating scale
CSHQ	children sleeping habit questionnaire
fMRI	functional magnetic resonance imaging
GABA	γ-aminobutyric acid
WHO	World Health Organization

Author details

Chuen Heung Yau*, Cheuk Long Ip, Yuk Yin Chau and Ho Cheung Lai
School of Chinese Medicine, Hong Kong Baptist University, Hong Kong

*Address all correspondence to: annyau33@yahoo.com.hk

References

[1] World Health Organization (WHO). Autism Spectrum Disorders: Fact Sheet. 2017. [Accessed: 21 May 2017]

[2] World Health Organization. The ICD-10 Classification of Mental and Behavioral Disorders: Clinical Descriptions and Diagnostic Guidelines. Geneva, Switzerland: World Health Organization; 1992

[3] American Psychiatric Association. Diagnostic and Statistical Manual of Mental Disorders. 5th ed. Washington, DC: American Psychiatric Publishing; 2013

[4] Hanson E, Kalish LA, Bunce E, Curtis C, McDaniel S, Ware J, et al. Use of complementary and alternative medicine among children diagnosed with autism spectrum disorder. Journal of Autism and Developmental Disorders. 2007;**37**(4):628-636

[5] Cheuk DKL, Wong V, Chen WX. Acupuncture for Autism Spectrum Disorders (ASD) (Review) The Cochrane Collaboration. Hoboken, N.J.: John Wiley and Sons, Ltd; 2011

[6] Kidd P. An approach to the nutritional management of autism. Alternative Therapies in Health and Medicine. 2003;**9**(5):24-61

[7] Ozonoff S, Heung K, Byrd R, Hansen R, Hertz-Picciotto I. The onset of autism: Patterns of symptom emergence in the first years of life. Autism Research. 2008;**1**(6):320-328

[8] Hoshino Y, Kaneko M, Yashima Y, Kumashiro H, Volkmar FR, Cohen DJ. Clinical features of autistic children with setback course in their infancy. Psychiatry and Clinical Neurosciences. 1987;**41**(2):237-245

[9] Samson AC, Phillips JM, Parker KJ, Shah S, Gross JJ, Hardan AY. Emotion dysregulation and the core features of autism spectrum disorder. Journal of Autism and Developmental Disorders. 2014;**44**(7):1766-1772

[10] Wood JJ, Gadow KD. Exploring the nature and function of anxiety in youth with autism spectrum disorders. Clinical Psychology: Science and Practice. 2010;**17**(4):281-292

[11] Kodak T, Piazza CC. Assessment and behavioral treatment of feeding and sleeping disorders in children with autism spectrum disorders. Child and Adolescent Psychiatric Clinics of North America. 2008;**17**(4):887-905

[12] Cohen S, Conduit R, Lockley SW, Rajaratnam SM, Cornish KM. The relationship between sleep and behavior in autism spectrum disorder (ASD): A review. Journal of Neurodevelopmental Disorders. 2014;**6**(1):44

[13] Harrington RA, Lee LC, Crum RM, Zimmerman AW, Hertz-Picciotto I. Serotonin hypothesis of autism: Implications for selective serotonin reuptake inhibitor use during pregnancy. Autism Research. 2013;**6**(3):149-168

[14] Lee EJ, Warden S. The effects of acupuncture on serotonin metabolism. European Journal of Integrative Medicine. 2016;**8**(4):355-367

[15] Jia HY, Li Q, Wang D. Scalp Acupuncture Therapy. 1st ed. Beijing, China: People's Medical Publishing House; 1994

[16] Yuan Q, Ma SL, Zhang JW. Effect of acupuncture on cerebral images in autism children. World Journal of Acupuncture and Moxibustion. 2004;**14**(3):3-8

[17] Nelson CA, Collins ML, MITCogNet. Handbook of Developmental Cognitive Neuroscience. Cambridge, Mass: MIT Press; 2001

[18] Domínguez PR. The study of postnatal and later development of the taste and olfactory systems using the human brain mapping approach: An update. Brain Research Bulletin. 2011;**84**(2):118-124

[19] Huttenlocher PR. Morphometric study of human cerebral cortex development. Neuropsychologia. 1990;**28**(6):517-527

[20] Comi AM, Zimmerman AW, Frye VH, Law PA, Peeden JN. Familial clustering of autoimmune disorders and evaluation of medical risk factors in autism. Journal of Child Neurology. 1999;**14**(6):388-394

[21] Sweeten TL, Bowyer SL, Posey DJ, Halberstadt GM, McDougle CJ. Increased prevalence of familial autoimmunity in probands with pervasive developmental disorders. Pediatrics. 2003;**112**(5):e420-e420

[22] Croen LA, Grether JK, Yoshida CK, Odouli R, Van de Water J. Maternal autoimmune diseases, asthma and allergies, and childhood autism spectrum disorders: A case-control study. Archives of Pediatrics & Adolescent Medicine. 2005;**159**(2):151-157

[23] Atladóttir HÓ, Pedersen MG, Thorsen P, Mortensen PB, Deleuran B, Eaton WW, et al. Association of family history of autoimmune diseases and autism spectrum disorders. Pediatrics. 2009;**124**(2):687-694

[24] Molloy CA, Morrow AL, Meinzen-Derr J, Dawson G, Bernier R, Dunn M, et al. Familial autoimmune thyroid disease as a risk factor for regression in children with autism spectrum disorder: A CPEA study. Journal of Autism and Developmental Disorders. 2006;**36**(3):317

[25] Potegal M, Kosorok MR, Davidson RJ. Temper tantrums in young children: 2. Tantrum duration and temporal organization. Journal of Developmental & Behavioral Pediatrics. 2003;**24**(3):148-154

[26] Potegal M, Carlson G, Margulies D, Gutkovitch Z, Wall M. Rages or temper tantrums? The behavioral organization, temporal characteristics, and clinical significance of angry-agitated outbursts in child psychiatry inpatients. Child Psychiatry and Human Development. 2009;**40**(4):621-636

[27] Stadler C, Sterzer P, Schmeck K, Krebs A, Kleinschmidt A, Poustka F. Reduced anterior cingulate activation in aggressive children and adolescents during affective stimulation: Association with temperament traits. Journal of Psychiatric Research. 2007;**41**(5):410-417

[28] Cho ZH, Hwang SC, Wong EK, Son YD, Kang CK, Park TS, et al. Neural substrates, experimental evidences and functional hypothesis of acupuncture mechanisms. Acta Neurologica Scandinavica. 2006;**113**(6):370-377

[29] Potegal M. Temporal and frontal lobe initiation and regulation of the top-down escalation of anger and aggression. Behavioural Brain Research. 2012;**231**(2):386-335

[30] Cortesi F, Giannotti F, Ivanenko A, Johnson K. Sleep in children with autistic spectrum disorder. Sleep Medicine. 2010;**11**(7):659-664

[31] Richdale AL, Schreck KA. Sleep problems in autism spectrum disorders: Prevalence, nature, & possible biopsychosocial aetiologies. Sleep Medicine Reviews. 2009;**13**(6):403-411

[32] Shergis JL, Ni X, Jackson ML, Zhang AL, Guo X, Li Y, et al. A systematic review of acupuncture for sleep quality in people with insomnia. Complementary Therapies in Medicine. 2016;**26**:11-20

Chapter 5

Stercobilin: A Putative Link between Autism and Gastrointestinal Distress?

Troy D. Wood, Amber Flynn Charlebois, Emily R. Sekera, Christopher L. Pennington, Heather L. Rudolph, Yong Seok Choi and Giuseppe Fanciulli

Abstract

Despite the increasing prevalence for its diagnosis in children, there are no clinical biomarkers of autism spectrum disorders (ASD). Herein a research journey is described that began by seeking evidence for the opioid excess theory of autism using mass spectrometry methods to screen human urine specimens and has evolved into the discovery of promising murine fecal biomarkers for ASD. Our results are consistent with an emerging body of evidence that shows that intestinal microflora from ASD subjects can be distinguished from controls, suggesting that metabolite differences due to the action of intestinal microbes may provide a means to identify ASD biomarkers.

Keywords: autism, biomarkers, stercobilin, mass spectrometry, metabolomics, microbiome

1. Introduction

Autism spectrum disorders (ASD) represent a group of neurobehavioral disorders first reported by Dr. Leo Kanner [1] which are characterized by impairments in social interactions, deficits in communications skills, repetitive behaviors, and other stereotypical behavioral patterns [2]. High rates of diagnosis in the United States (up to 1 in 59 children) [3] exemplify the seriousness of ASD as a medical concern. There is great interest in identifying potential ASD biomarkers, as the evidence indicates that early diagnosis and intervention leads to improved long-term outcomes for individuals with ASD [4, 5]. While considerable effort has been dedicated toward discovering potential genetic factors associated with ASD, it is becoming increasingly clear that genetic factors alone are insufficient to explain overall ASD etiology [6]. Combined, these factors have inhibited the development of a grand unified theory (GUT) for autism [7] (note: the irony that gut microbiota may be an important factor contributing to a GUT of ASD is not lost upon the authors).

While a GUT for ASD may be unrealistic because of heterogeneity in causation and severity, increasing attention has been devoted toward identifying potential metabolic molecular markers of ASD. One approach has been to consider conditions that are comorbid with ASD, in particular, gastrointestinal distress, which is a

IntechOpen

condition observed in a high percentage of persons with ASD [8–10]. Interestingly, the homeostasis of the central nervous system (CNS) is regulated by the gut microbiome [11, 12], and furthermore the microbiome is known to have effects in neuropsychiatric disorders [13, 14]. Therefore, the effects of the microbiome on the gut-brain axis are a potentially promising source for metabolic biomarker discovery for ASD.

In this chapter, we will cover our combined efforts to discover potential ASD biomarkers. While we initially explored the possibility that peptides consistent with the opioid excess theory of ASD [15] may possess diagnostic value, our search took a new direction during the course of research. Our results are discussed within the context of our results alongside other research that shows distinctions in the microbiota of subjects with ASD *vs.* controls.

2. The opioid excess theory of autism

Anecdotally, two of the authors of this chapter had observed substantial behavioral improvements in family members who had been diagnosed with childhood autism or were exhibiting symptoms of ASD when their diets were altered to avoid milk (casein) and/or wheat (gluten), known now as the gluten-free casein-free (GFCF) diet [16–18]. Therefore, our journey delving into the etiology of ASD initially involved an exploration into the idea of increased intestinal permeability [19], also referred to as the "leaky gut syndrome." This syndrome describes the passage of potentially bioactive peptides, created from the incomplete breakdown of the proteins through the intestinal membrane, into the blood stream and ultimately into the brain through the blood-brain barrier (BBB) [20–23]. The combined work of Panksepp [15], Shattock [17, 18, 24, 25], Waring [26], Gardner [27], and Reichelt [28] caused us to pursue this area of research. Now termed the opioid excess theory, this invaluable research from the 1990s and early 2000s explains how some of the incompletely metabolized protein pieces are described and compared to endogenous opioids, β-endorphins. An outstanding account of the opioid excess theory has been described and is highly recommended [29].

3. Transition from the opioid excess theory to potential biomarkers

Our research into ASD biomarkers began by testing the biological effects of administration of gluten exorphins (GEs) to rodents and by developing methodology to detect opioid peptides in biological fluids. Our work was inspired along two avenues. The first inspiration was derived from the results of Fukudome et al. who showed that in animal models, GE-B5 stimulated glucose-induced insulin release after intragastric administration [30]. The second inspiration was derived from the intriguing results of the Reichelt group [28], who had demonstrated that dietary intervention to eliminate casein and gluten from the diet in individuals with ASD led to improvements in the use of social, cognitive, and communicative skills over a period of 4 years.

The Sassari, Italy, experiments were performed to test whether GEs could elicit biological activity in rats. Intracerebroventricular (ICV)-injection of gluten exorphin B5 into rats stimulated the release of prolactin through activation of opioid receptors [31, 32]. Subsequently, efforts to determine the site of action of GE-B5 on prolactin secretion were conducted by pretreating male rats with naloxone methobromide (NMB), an opioid antagonist that does not cross the BBB [33]; NMB preadministration completely abolished the prolactin response. These results indicated that GE-B5 stimulates prolactin secretion through opioid receptors located outside the BBB. Since opioid peptides do not exert their effect on prolactin secretion directly, but via a reduced dopaminergic response, these data suggested that GE-B5 modifies brain neurotransmitter release without crossing the BBB. These results clearly demonstrated that GE-B5 could elicit opioid activity in rats. Interestingly, GE-B4, whose structure (Tyr-Gly-Gly-Trp) is identical to that of the NH_2-terminal sequence of GE-B5, did not elicit such activity, thus suggesting that the presence of the carboxyl-terminal leucine in GE-B5 is essential for its action on prolactin secretion [34].

In a series of papers published between our groups at Sassari and Buffalo, we developed approaches to detect GEs in biological fluids using liquid chromatography-mass spectrometry (LC-MS) methods. First, we used LC-MS to detect GE-A5 in sheep cerebrospinal fluid (CSF) [35]. Next, using a slightly different protocol, we developed LC-MS for the detection of GE-B5 in CSF and recognized that stability was a significant issue; in the absence of protease inhibitors, GE-B5 degraded more than 50% within 600 min after collection [36]. Thus, when methods were developed for the detection of GEs in human blood plasma, aprotinin, a protease inhibitor, was added to plasma samples from patients with celiac disease (CD), a genetic autoimmune disease which induces inflammation to patients' small intestine by their ingestion of gluten. CD patients consumed a pizza made from wheat gluten, and their blood was collected at intervals over a 120 min period. Using liquid chromatography-tandem mass spectrometry (LC-MS/MS), GE-B4 and GE-B5 were detected in three of four patients with CD, the first time GEs were detected in human blood [37]. An LC-MS/MS spectrum of GE-B5 in blood plasma collected from a CD patient 90 min after consumption of pizza containing wheat gluten flour is shown in **Figure 1**. However, GE-B4 and GE-B5 were detected in the blood plasma of two of the four patients before consuming the pizza, indicating another potential dietary source for the GEs.

Although we had established that GEs were detectable in human blood, their rapid degradation in the absence of protease inhibitors led us to become skeptical that GEs would contribute to the opioid excess theory of ASD in a substantive way, especially after the report that indicated no significant differences in the high-performance liquid chromatography (HPLC) urinary profiles of the children with ASD and controls and no detection of GEs in the urine specimens by matrix-assisted laser desorption/ionization (MALDI) mass spectrometry [38]. Urine had shown some promise as a specimen that might harbor biomarkers of diagnostic value for ASD [20, 39]. In our own research, serendipity had a hand yet to play, and it led to a new viewpoint. GE-B5, one of the target exorphins, produces a $[M+H]^+$ ion at *m/z* 595, with the distinct fragmentation pattern as shown in **Figure 1**. We had

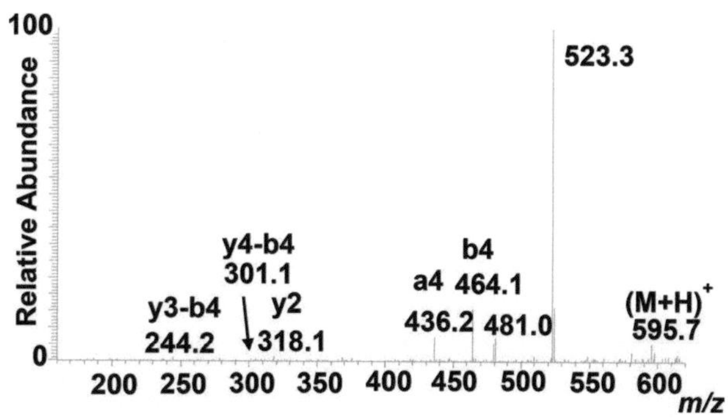

Figure 1.
LC-MS/MS of GE-B5 detected in a sample of human blood plasma taken from a CD patient 90 min after consumption of wheat gluten flour pizza, from [37].

begun using LC-MS/MS to screen for GEs, and other potential opiate peptides, in urine. Using specimens from urines collected and reported in [38], we observed by LC-MS/MS a significant difference in the abundance of a species with *m/z* 595 in the urine specimens between ASD and controls.

As shown in **Figure 2**, the LC chromatograms of (A) control and (B) ASD urines show a remarkable difference in abundance for this species which elutes at ~12.9 min; typical depletion in ASD urines was 67% vs. the controls (in **Figure 2B** depletion is a factor of 68). The MS/MS of this species, codenamed "595A" at the time, is shown in **Figure 2C**. Clearly, the fragmentation pattern of 595A does not correspond to that of GE-B5 shown in **Figure 1** and is dominated by the formation of two product ions at *m/z* 470 and *m/z* 345, respectively. While we did not know the identity of 595A initially, intuition about fragmentation behavior of small molecules led us to suspect a particularly stable molecule, perhaps of the porphyrin family. The emergence of the Human Metabolome Database (HMDB) in 2007 [40] allowed us to search for possible metabolites, and we obtained one hit that satisfied the *m/z* of 595A and porphyrin metabolic pathways—L-stercobilin, $C_{33}H_{46}N_4O_6$, a metabolite found in mammalian waste products. Subsequently, we purchased stercobilin hydrochloride from Frontier Scientific and performed nanoelectrospray ionization (nanoESI) and MS/MS on stercobilin hydrochloride and obtained the same fragmentation pattern [41], and we have established this identity in a number of publications [42–45]. We had thus identified 595A as L-stercobilin as a potential biomarker of ASD in human urine. However, methods of performing reliable

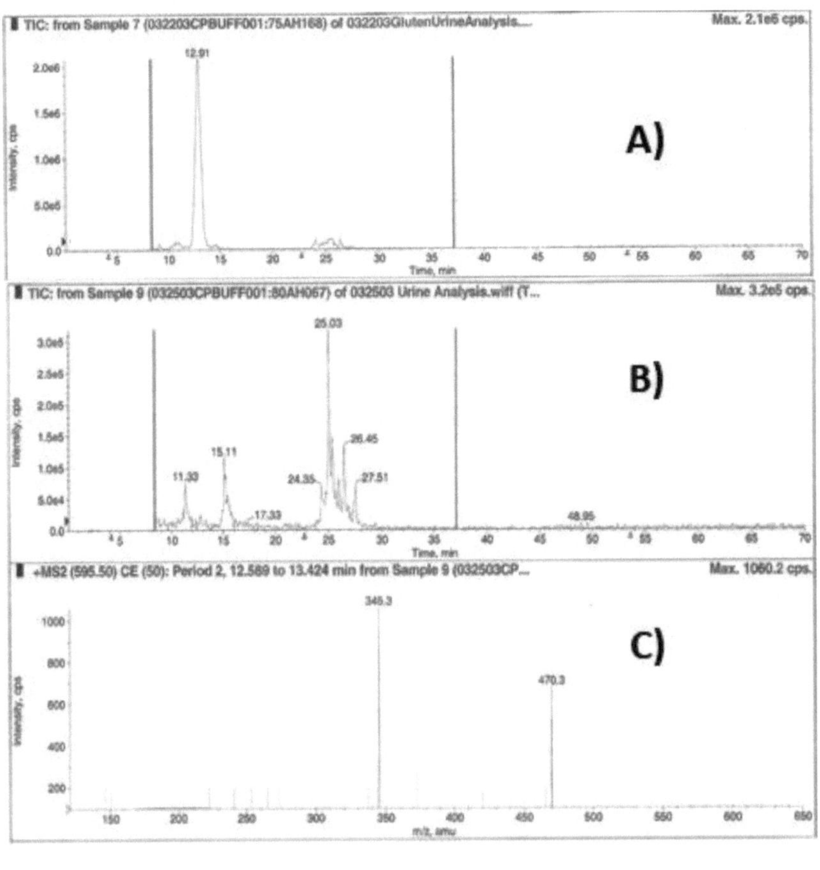

Figure 2.
Chromatogram of (A) control urine extract and (B) ASD urine extract. (C) MS/MS of the peak at 12.9 min in the ASD urine extract, with a precursor ion mass of m/z 595.

quantification were needed in order to validate whether this was the case; unfortunately, isotopically labeled standards of stercobilin are not commercially available. Thus, we embarked on approaches to synthesize a suitable label for stercobilin that could be used as an internal standard for mass spectrometry analysis.

4. Strategies for producing tetrapyrrole standards

4.1 Methyl esterification of bilins

In order to test whether stercobilin (or any other tetrapyrrole bilin) might be useful as a potential ASD biomarker, it would be necessary to have a reliable standard for quantitative purposes. Our first approach to develop a standard for the bilins was to perform methyl esterification [42]. To achieve methyl esterification of bilins, methanolic HCl was first prepared by the combination of 160 μL of acetyl chloride with 1 mL of anhydrous methanol dropwise *slowly*. Next, 10 μg of the bilin was dissolved in 500 μL of the methanolic HCl and reacted at room temperature for 2 h. This led to efficient (>90%), but incomplete, derivatization of stercobilin at its carboxyl groups to the dimethylester; MS/MS using collision-induced dissociation (CID) with argon gas confirmed that derivatization occurs at each carboxyl group, and although most of the bilins were converted to the dimethylester form, a small amount of the monomethyl ester was also produced. Furthermore, the dimethylesters were found to have high solubility in 50/50 methanol/water; this was found to be problematic for long-term stability, as the level of esterification would decrease over storage time at 4°C.

4.2 ^{18}O labeling of bilins

In another attempt to quantitate stercobilin, an isotopologue standard was created based off of the work by Bergmann et al. [46]. Isotopologues are often ideal internal standards for quantitation using mass spectrometry because the isotopologue is itself chemically similar to the analyte of interest but is shifted in mass due to the incorporation of another isotope. In the structure of stercobilin, the four oxygens within the carboxylic acid groups on the inner pyrroles are labile and able to be exchanged with the oxygen atoms of $H_2{}^{18}O$ (as can be seen in red in **Figure 3**). The reaction works under an acidic environment utilizing trifluoroacetic acid (TFA) as a proton donor to aid in the protonation of the carbonyl oxygen for the nucleophilic substitution reaction. Currently, we have scaled up our original procedure [47] by using ca. 5×10^{-6} mol of stercobilin mixed with 10 μL 5% (v/v) TFA and 95 μL of $H_2{}^{18}O$ in an LC autosampler vial with screw cap lid. The vial is placed in an incubator at 70°C for 8 h [43]. Following the reaction, the sample is dried down under air and reconstituted in 100 mL of 20:80 (v/v) ACN/H_2O.

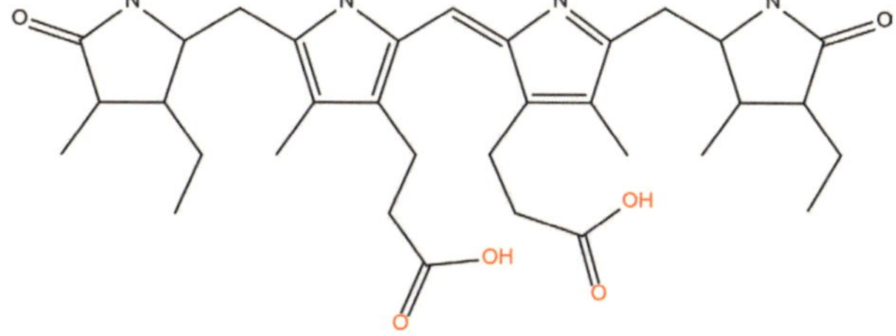

Figure 3.
The structure of stercobilin with the labile oxygen sites highlighted in red.

m/z peak ($^{18}O_n$)	% labeling
595 ($^{18}O_0$)	0.16 ± 0.04
597 ($^{18}O_1$)	7.2 ± 0.9
599 ($^{18}O_2$)	25.6 ± 0.8
601 ($^{18}O_3$)	38.6 ± 0.7
603 ($^{18}O_4$)	28.5 ± 0.5

Table 1.
Corresponding m/z peaks from labeled stercobilin with the percentage of labeling of each peak denoted.

To improve upon our previous ^{18}O-stercobilin isotopologue yield, the reaction was conducted at a higher temperature [47] than what was reported by Bergmann et al. [46]. To further push the reaction toward full labeling, the reaction is carried out a second time under the same initial conditions except for allowing it to react for 22 h instead of 8. With this a labeling efficiency of 72.1 ± 0.3% was observed with minimal original stercobilin left in the reaction (**Table 1**). The results of this experiment have allowed for the quantitation of stercobilin within fecal samples.

4.3 Deuterated stercobilin

Next, we synthesized a more stable isotopologue of stercobilin through the use of deuterium-carbon bonds, which were achieved by the incorporation of deuterium across several of the carbon-carbon double bonds of bilirubin as described by Putzbach et al. [48]. This protocol incorporated deuterium atoms into bilirubin affording stercobilin with a mass increase of more than 12 atomic mass units. The conversion of bilirubin to stercobilin was previously reported (**Figure 4**) [49].

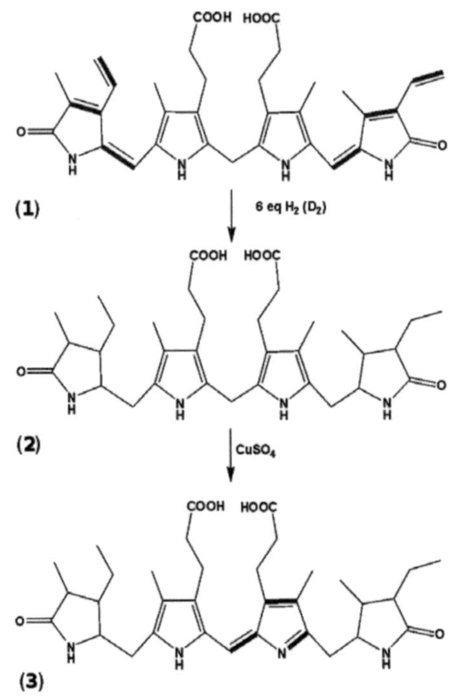

Figure 4.
Step (1) involves the reduction of bilirubin into stercobilinogen. Step (2) involves partial oxidation of stercobilinogen into stercobilin (3), our desired product.

This method allowed us to reduce the six non-pyrrole C = C double bonds with hydrogen gas (control reaction) or with deuterium gas (isotopologue) producing stercobilinogen and labeled stercobilinogen, respectively [44, 50]. For the deuterated isotopologue, bilirubin (200 mg) was combined with 25 mL deuterated glacial acetic acid (CD_3COOD) and 200 mg of palladium on carbon, and deuteration was allowed to proceed for 1.5 h at 65°C to produce stercobilinogen. Stercobilinogen is subsequently aerated in the presence of copper sulfate, resulting in the final product, stercobilin. Combined nuclear magnetic resonance (NMR) and MS/MS analysis indicated incorporation of deuterium at all 12 sites, with no evidence of unreacted bilirubin.

5. Biomarker validation: connection to the microbiome

Utilizing the ^{18}O isotopologue standard, the amount of stercobilin could be quantified within the fecal samples of a murine model of ASD. In the described study, a population of mice with Timothy Syndrome (TS) was utilized; these mice have been previously described as exhibiting autistic behaviors. In particular, the mice used herein had a more severe case of TS, TS2-NEO, caused by a missense mutation in exon 8 at G406R in tandem with a flipped neomycin cassette, allowing for the mice to survive to adulthood [51]. Fourteen pairs of mice that were age- and gender-matched were utilized in this study.

Response factor calculations were first completed in order to quantify the amount of labeled stercobilin in the fecal samples as well as account for the amount of unlabeled stercobilin that would be present in the sample from the isotopologue standard. Calculations of the concentration of stercobilin were determined utilizing the *m/z* 601 peak from the labeled stock. Concentrations were then normalized per gram of fecal material. From these calculations, box and whisker plots were created and are shown in **Figure 5** for both stercobilin and its precursor, stercobilinogen. An unpaired *t*-test was utilized to determine *p*-values and to establish whether the populations' mean bilin levels were statistically significantly different, or not, from each other.

When calculating the average moles of stercobilin utilizing the peak area of the *m/z* of 601 of WT and TS2-NEO populations, values of $1.84 \times 10^{-8} \pm 7.1 \times 10^{-9}$ and $9.59 \times 10^{-9} \pm 4.1 \times 10^{-9}$ mol/g feces were found for the two populations, respectively. These values show a depletion of ca. 48% in stercobilin levels of TS2-NEO mice ($p \leq 0.001$). In comparison, calculating the average moles of stercobilinogen utilizing the peak area of the *m/z* of 601 of WT and TS2-NEO populations, values of $1.13 \times 10^{-8} \pm 1.1 \times 10^{-8}$ and $5.55 \times 10^{-9} \pm 3.7 \times 10^{-9}$ mol/g feces were found for the two populations, respectively. These values showed a depletion of 51% in

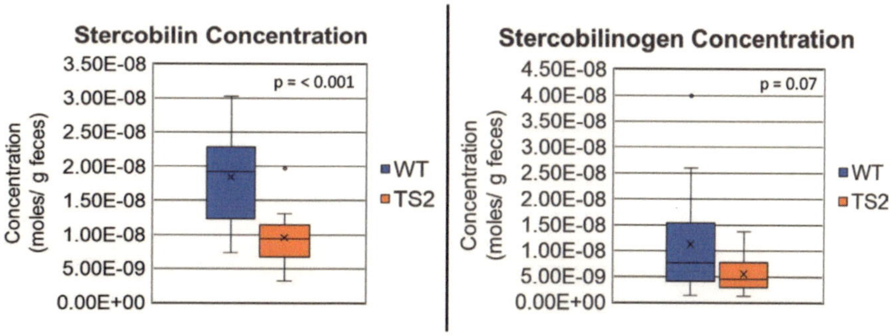

Figure 5.
A comparison of the average concentration of both stercobilin and stercobilinogen found in wild type (WT) as opposed to mice with TS2-NEO per gram of fecal material. The p-values calculated from the unpaired t-test are shown in the upper right-hand corner of the box and whisker plots.

stercobilinogen levels of TS2-NEO mice ($p = 0.07$). A larger sample set will be necessary to determine the significance of depletion in stercobilinogen. Furthermore, the p-values determined were improved upon since our last report with a study of nine pairs of mice [43].

The depletion of stercobilin in the ASD model of mice relative to controls at a greater than 99.9% confidence level suggests that stercobilin depletion in fecal material may have potential value as a biomarker for ASD in humans. Although less statistically significant, stercobilinogen, the metabolic precursor to stercobilin, is also depleted in fecal samples. The observation of these depletions suggests that there may be interference in the metabolic pathway that allows for the differences. As shown in **Figure 6**, stercobilin and stercobilinogen are products of heme catabolism. As bilirubin glucuronides enter the intestines, the action of enzyme systems by anaerobic bacterial flora converts the glucuronides to mesobilirubinogen, which is further converted to stercobilinogen.

Our results are also intriguing in the context of a discovery decades ago by Gustafsson and Lanke in which they observed no bilins present in the feces or urine of germfree rats [52]. Once the germfree animals were exposed to fecal matter from control animals, they too began to produce bilins to the same extent as the controls (when both groups were given identical diets). Moreover, they observed that the negative urobilin test (note: urobilin is a metabolic product derived from urobilinogen and is primarily excreted through urine, as shown in **Figure 6**) turned positive in germfree animals infected with a single *Clostridium*-like microorganism that had been isolated from the intestinal contents of rats that showed the presence of bilins in fecal matter. The bilin output increased in these animals after infection

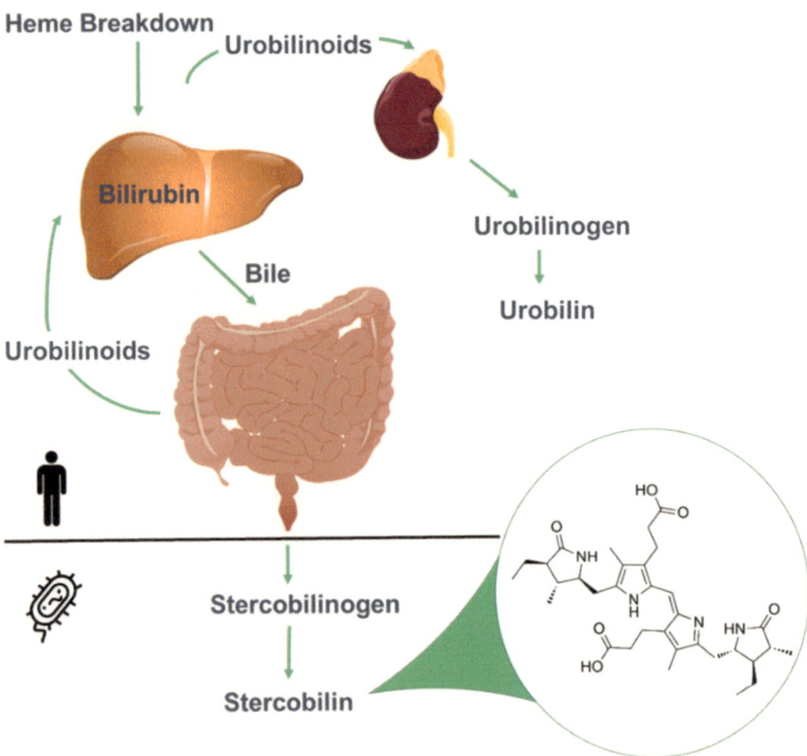

Figure 6.
A depiction of the catabolism of heme into stercobilin. The enterohepatic cycle in which stercobilin can be recirculated back and excreted instead through the urine is also shown. The line shows the point in which bacterial interaction takes over in the metabolic pathway to create stercobilin.

with *Escherichia coli*, although not reaching the levels observed for controls [52]. In context, our results showing depleted stercobilin and stercobilinogen in fecal matter of ASD model mice might suggest that *Clostridium* constitutes part of their microbiota but that *E. coli* may have been impacted such that bilin production is reduced. Clearly, microbiological testing of fecal matter from ASD model mice is needed to provide additional insight. A recent report on microbiota and fecal metabolites comparing humans with ASD *vs.* controls revealed discernible differences between the two groups [53]. How this might be applicable to our murine ASD model is a subject worthy of follow-up investigation.

Due to the high number of differences observed in the gut microbiome of those with ASD [54], it is possible that the bacterial population variations are making an important impact on bilin metabolism. The significance of the gut on brain activity has begun to be heavily researched. In some studies, disorders such as autism, depression, and anxiety have seen lessening of symptoms based on the introduction of different bacteria within the patient's microbiome [13]. In particular, the altered microbiome of those with ASD has developed changes in the production of short-chain fatty acids. One such fatty acid noted was propionic acid, which has been reported to be increased in those with autism [55]. Activity on propionic acid chains are important to the conversion of bilirubin to bilirubin diglucuronide and may provide insight into the potential depletion observed [56].

Based on previous knowledge of the production of stercobilin within humans, the results presented herein suggest that microbiome analysis coupled to the molecular analysis of bilins from fecal material is warranted. Fecal material can be collected noninvasively and proved to give a wealth of metabolomic information. Through the combination of these techniques, a combinatory biochemical and molecular biological approach to diagnosing ASD may yet be developed.

6. Conclusions

The discovery that stercobilin, and to a lesser extent stercobilinogen, are depleted in the fecal matter from a murine ASD model gives promise of the potential of these substances to serve as clinical biomarkers for ASD. Work to understand the relationship between the depletion of these bilins and the identity of the microbiota responsible is intriguing, as is the possibility that microbiota may play a role in the etiology of ASD; if this is true, it means that fecal transplants may have impact in the treatment of ASD, as recent clinical evidence suggests [57].

Acknowledgements

The authors would like to thank all of their coworkers who contributed to the results described in this chapter, including Kevin Quinn, Charmion Cruickshank-Quinn, Jordan Coffey, Anthony Vadas, Thomas Puleo, Katelyn Lewis, Gregory Pirrone, Eric Helms, Alessandra Dettori, Emanuela Azara, Mauro Marchetti, Paolo Tomasi, Giuseppe Delitala, Emma Fenude, Maria Piera Demontis, Elisabetta Alberico, Vittorio Anania, Silvia Gianorso, Will Friesen, Nhu Nguyen-Dudziak, Stephen Carro, and Michael Wach. Financial support for this research has come from the United Kingdom Legal Services Commission, the Fondazione Banco di Sardegna, the California Scottish Rite, the Mark Diamond Research Fund, and the National Institutes of Health through the Center for Research Resources (Grant #S10-RR029517).

Conflict of interest

Troy Wood receives royalties from sales of his textbook from TopHat (Toronto, Canada). No other authors have any conflict of interest.

Author details

Troy D. Wood[1*], Amber Flynn Charlebois[2], Emily R. Sekera[1], Christopher L. Pennington[3], Heather L. Rudolph[4], Yong Seok Choi[5] and Giuseppe Fanciulli[6]

1 Department of Chemistry, University at Buffalo, Buffalo, NY, United States

2 Department of Chemistry, Nazareth College, Rochester, NY, United States

3 Shared Equipment Authority, Rice University, Houston, TX, United States

4 Thermo Fisher Scientific, Grand Island, NY, United States

5 College of Pharmacy, Dankook University, Cheonon, Chungnam, Republic of Korea

6 Department of Medical, Surgical and Experimental Sciences, University of Sassari, Sassari, Sardinia, Italy

*Address all correspondence to: twood@buffalo.edu

References

[1] Kanner L, Eisenberg L. Early infantile autism, 1943-1955. Psychiatric research reports of the American Psychiatric Association. 1957;7:55-65

[2] Association AP. Diagnostic and Statistical Manual of Mental Disorders. 5th ed. Arlington, VA: American Psychiatric Association; 2013

[3] Baio J, Wiggins L, Christensen DL, Maenner MJ, Daniels J, Warren Z, et al. Prevalence of autism spectrum disorder among children aged 8 years—Autism and developmental disabilities monitoring network, 11 sites, United States, 2014. MMWR Surveillance Summaries. 2018;**67**(6):1-23

[4] Ospina MB, Krebs Seida J, Clark B, Karkhaneh M, Hartling L, Tjosvold L, et al. Behavioural and developmental interventions for autism spectrum disorder: A clinical systematic review. PLoS One. 2008;**3**(11):e3755

[5] Ozonoff S, Goodlin-Jones BL, Solomon M. Evidence-based assessment of autism spectrum disorders in children and adolescents. Journal of Clinical Child and Adolescent Psychology. 2005;**34**(3):523-540

[6] Herbert MR, Russo JP, Yang S, Roohi J, Blaxill M, Kahler SG, et al. Autism and environmental genomics. Neurotoxicology. 2006;**27**(5):671-684

[7] Rudolph HL, Friesen WL, Wood TD. The hunt for biomarkers of autism spectrum disorders. Journal of Metabolomics & Systems Biology. 2013;**1**(1):1-11

[8] Bauman ML. Medical comorbidities in autism: Challenges to diagnosis and treatment. Neurotherapeutics. 2010;**7**(3):320-327

[9] Kohane IS, McMurry A, Weber G, MacFadden D, Rappaport L, Kunkel L, et al. The co-morbidity burden of children and young adults with autism spectrum disorders. PLoS One. 2012;**7**(4):e33224

[10] Bresnahan M, Hornig M, Schultz AF, Gunnes N, Hirtz D, Lie KK, et al. Association of maternal report of infant and toddler gastrointestinal symptoms with autism: Evidence from a prospective birth cohort. JAMA Psychiatry. 2015;**72**(5):466-474

[11] Rhee SH, Pothoulakis C, Mayer EA. Principles and clinical implications of the brain-gut-enteric microbiota axis. Nature Reviews. Gastroenterology & Hepatology. 2009;**6**(5):306-314

[12] Sherwin E, Sandhu KV, Dinan TG, Cryan JF. May the force be with you: The light and dark sides of the microbiota-gut-brain axis in neuropsychiatry. CNS Drugs. 2016;**30**(11):1019-1041

[13] Cryan JF, Dinan TG. Mind-altering microorganisms: The impact of the gut microbiota on brain and behaviour. Nature Reviews. Neuroscience. 2012;**13**(10):701-712

[14] Rogers GB, Keating DJ, Young RL, Wong ML, Licinio J, Wesselingh S. From gut dysbiosis to altered brain function and mental illness: Mechanisms and pathways. Molecular Psychiatry. 2016;**21**(6):738-748

[15] Panksepp J. A neurochemical theory of autism. Trends in Neurosciences. 1979;**2**:174-177

[16] Whiteley P, Shattock P, Knivsberg AM, Seim A, Reichelt KL, Todd L, et al. Gluten- and casein-free dietary intervention for autism spectrum conditions. Frontiers in Human Neuroscience. 2012;**6**:344

[17] Whiteley P, Rodgers J, Savery D, Shattock P. A gluten-free diet as an

intervention for autism and associated spectrum disorders: Preliminary findings. Autism. 1999;**3**:45-65

[18] Whiteley P, Haracopos D, Knivsberg AM, Reichelt KL, Parlar S, Jacobsen J, et al. The ScanBrit randomised, controlled, single-blind study of a gluten- and casein-free dietary intervention for children with autism spectrum disorders. Nutritional Neuroscience. 2010;**13**(2):87-100

[19] Arrieta MC, Bistritz L, Meddings JB. Alterations in intestinal permeability. Gut. 2006;**55**(10):1512-1520

[20] Alcorn A, Berney T, Bretherton K, Mills M, Savery D, Shattock P. Urinary compounds in autism. Journal of Intellectual Disability Research. 2004;**48**(Pt 3):274-278

[21] Gillberg C, Terenius L, Lonnerholm G. Endorphin activity in childhood psychosis. Spinal fluid levels in 24 cases. Archives of General Psychiatry. 1985;**42**:780-783

[22] Cazzullo AG, Musetti MC, Musetti L, Bajo S, Sacerdote P, Panerai A. Beta-endorphin levels in peripheral blood mononuclear cells and long-term naltrexone treatment in autistic children. European Neuropsychopharmacology. 1999;**9**:361-366

[23] Nelson KB, Grether JK, Croen LA, Dambrosia JM, Dickens BF, Jelliffe LL, et al. Neuropeptides and neurotrophins in neonatal blood of children with autism or mental retardation. Annals of Neurology. 2001;**49**(5):597-606

[24] Shattock P, Kennedy A, Rowell F, Berney T. Role of neuropeptides in autism and their relationship with classical neurotransmitters. Brain Dysfunction. 1990;**3**:328-345

[25] Shattock P, Lowdon G. Proteins, peptides and autism. Part 2: Implications for the education and care of people with autism. Brain Dysfunction. 1991;**4**:323-334

[26] Waring RH, Klovrza LV. Sulphur metabolism in autism. Journal of Environmental Medicine. 2000;**10**:25-32

[27] Gardner ML. Intestinal assimilation of intact peptides and proteins from the diet—A neglected field? Biological Reviews of the Cambridge Philosophical Society. 1984;**59**(3):289-331

[28] Knivsberg AM, Reichelt KL, N⊘dland M, H⊘ien T. Autistic syndromes and diet: A follow-up study. Scandinavian Journal of Educational Research. 1995;**39**(3):223-236

[29] Whiteley P, Shattock P. Biochemical aspects in autism spectrum disorders: Updating the opioid-excess theory and presenting new opportunities for biomedical intervention. Expert Opinion on Therapeutic Targets. 2002;**6**(2):175-183

[30] Fukudome S, Shimatsu A, Suganuma H, Yoshikawa M. Effect of gluten exorphins A5 and B5 on the postprandial plasma insulin level in conscious rats. Life Sciences. 1995;**57**(7):729-734

[31] Fanciulli G, Dettori A, Tomasi PA, Demontis MP, Gianorso S, Anania V, et al. Prolactin and growth hormone response to intracerebroventricular administration of the food opioid peptide gluten exorphin B5 in rats. Life Sciences. 2002;**71**(20):2383-2390

[32] Fanciulli G, Dettori A, Fenude E, Demontis MP, Alberico E, Delitala G, et al. Intravenous administration of the food-derived opioid peptide gluten exorphin B5 stimulates prolactin secretion in rats. Pharmacological Research. 2003;**47**(1):53-58

[33] Fanciulli G, Dettori A, Demontis MP, Tomasi PA, Anania V, Delitala G. Gluten exorphin B5 stimulates prolactin secretion through opioid receptors located outside the blood-brain barrier. Life Sciences. 2005;**76**(15):1713-1719

[34] Fanciulli G, Dettori A, Demontis MP, Anania V, Delitala G. Serum prolactin levels after administration of the alimentary opioid peptide gluten exorphin B4 in male rats. Nutritional Neuroscience. 2004;**7**(1):53-55

[35] Fanciulli G, Azara E, Wood TD, Dettori A, Delitala G, Marchetti M. Quantification of gluten exorphin A5 in cerebrospinal fluid by liquid chromatography-mass spectrometry. Journal of Chromatography. B, Analytical Technologies in the Biomedical and Life Sciences. 2006;**833**(2):204-209

[36] Fanciulli G, Azara E, Wood TD, Delitala G, Marchetti M. Liquid chromatography-mass spectrometry assay for quantification of gluten exorphin B5 in cerebrospinal fluid. Journal of Chromatography. B, Analytical Technologies in the Biomedical and Life Sciences. 2007;**852**(1-2):485-490

[37] Pennington CL, Dufresne CP, Fanciulli G, Wood TD. Detection of gluten exorphin B4 and B5 in human blood by liquid chromatography-mass spectrometry/mass spectrometry. Open Spectroscopy Journal. 2007;**1**(1):9-16

[38] Cass H, Gringras P, March J, McKendrick I, O'Hare AE, Owen L, et al. Absence of urinary opioid peptides in children with autism. Archives of Disease in Childhood. 2008;**93**(9):745-750

[39] Bull G, Shattock P, Whiteley P, Anderson R, Groundwater PW, Lough JW, et al. Indolyl-3-acryloylglycine (IAG) is a putative diagnostic urinary marker for autism spectrum disorders. Medical Science Monitor. 2003;**9**(10):CR422-CR425

[40] Wishart DS, Tzur D, Knox C, Eisner R, Guo AC, Young N, et al. HMDB: The human metabolome database. Nucleic Acids Research. 2007;**35**(Database):D521-D526

[41] Wood TD, Pennington CL, Choi YS, editors. Stercobilin: A possible biomarker for autism? In: Proc 55th ASMS Conf on Mass Spectrometry & Allied Topics; 2007 June 3-7, 2007; Indianapolis, IN

[42] Quinn KD, Nguyen NQ , Wach MM, Wood TD. Tandem mass spectrometry of bilin tetrapyrroles by electrospray ionization and collision-induced dissociation. Rapid Communications in Mass Spectrometry. 2012;**26**(16):1767-1775

[43] Sekera ER, Rudolph HL, Carro SD, Morales MJ, Bett GCL, Rasmusson RL, et al. Depletion of stercobilin in fecal matter from a mouse model of autism spectrum disorders. Metabolomics. 2017;**13**(11):132

[44] Coffey JM, Vadas AJ, Puleo TR, Lewis KP, Pirrone GF, Rudolph HL, et al. Synthesis and characterization of a deuterium labeled stercobilin: A potential biomarker for autism. Journal of Labelled Compounds and Radiopharmaceuticals. 2018;**61**(10): 742-748

[45] Sekera ER, Wood TD. Examination of the fragmentation behavior of hemin and bilin tetrapyrroles by electrospray ionization and collision-induced dissociation. Mass Spectrometry Letters. 2018;**9**:91-94

[46] Bergmann D, Hubner F, Humpf HU. Stable isotope dilution analysis of small molecules with carboxylic acid functions using 18O labeling for HPLC-ESI-MS/MS: Analysis of fumonisin B1. Journal of Agricultural and Food Chemistry. 2013;**61**(33):7904-7908

[47] Rudolph HL, Sekera ER, Wood TD. Stable (18) O-labeling method for stercobilin and other bilins for metabolomics. Rapid Communications in Mass Spectrometry. 2016;**30**(13):1469-1474

[48] Putzbach K, Krucker M, Albert K, Grusak MA, Tang G, Dolnikowski GG. Structure determination of partially deuterated carotenoids from intrinsically labeled vegetables by HPLC-MS and 1H NMR. Journal of Agricultural and Food Chemistry. 2005;**53**(3):671-677

[49] Kay IT, Weimer M, Watson CJ. The formation in vitro of stercobilin from bilirubin. The Journal of Biological Chemistry. 1963;**238**:1122-1123

[50] Rohwedder WK, Scholfield CR, Rakoff H, Nowakowska J, Dutton HJ. Infrared analysis of methyl stearates containing deuterium. Analytical Chemistry. 1967;**39**(7):820

[51] Bader PL, Faizi M, Kim LH, Owen SF, Tadross MR, Alfa RW, et al. Mouse model of timothy syndrome recapitulates triad of autistic traits. Proceedings of the National Academy of Sciences of the United States of America. 2011;**108**(37):15432-15437

[52] Gustafsson BE, Lanke LS. Bilirubin and urobilins in germfree, ex-germfree, and conventional rats. The Journal of Experimental Medicine. 1960;**112**:975-981

[53] Kang DW, Ilhan ZE, Isern NG, Hoyt DW, Howsmon DP, Shaffer M, et al. Differences in fecal microbial metabolites and microbiota of children with autism spectrum disorders. Anaerobe. 2018;**49**:121-131

[54] Ding HT, Taur Y, Walkup JT. Gut microbiota and autism: Key concepts and findings. Journal of Autism and Developmental Disorders. 2017;**47**(2):480-489

[55] Wang L, Christophersen CT, Sorich MJ, Gerber JP, Angley MT, Conlon MA. Elevated fecal short chain fatty acid and ammonia concentrations in children with autism spectrum disorder. Digestive Diseases and Sciences. 2012;**57**(8):2096-2102

[56] Gossauer A. Synthesis of bilins. In: Kadish KM, Smith KM, Guilard R, editors. The Porphyrin Handbook. 13. Vol. 84. San Diego: Academic Press; 2003. pp. 237-274

[57] Kang DW, Adams JB, Gregory AC, Borody T, Chittick L, Fasano A, et al. Microbiota transfer therapy alters gut ecosystem and improves gastrointestinal and autism symptoms: An open-label study. Microbiome. 2017;**5**(1):10